Thin Within

Thin Within

A Grace-Oriented Approach
To Lasting Weight Loss

Judy Wardell Halliday, R.N.
Arthur W. Halliday, M.D.

with Heidi Bylsma
Illustrated by Sally Rackets

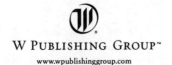

W PUBLISHING GROUP™
www.wpublishinggroup.com
A Division of Thomas Nelson, Inc.
www.ThomasNelson.com

Every effort has been made to ensure that the information contained in this book is complete and accurate. However, neither the publisher nor the authors are engaged in rendering professional advice or services to the individual reader. The ideas, procedures, and suggestions contained in this book are not intended as a substitute for consulting with your physician. All matters regarding your health require medical supervision. Neither the authors nor the publisher shall be liable or responsible for any loss, injury, or damage allegedly arising from any information or suggestions in this book. The opinions expressed in this book represent the personal views of the authors and not of the publisher.

Published by W Publishing Group, a Division of Thomas Nelson, Inc., P.O. Box 141000, Nashville, Tennessee 37214.

Interior Illustrations by Sally Rackets.

Unless otherwise indicated, Scripture quotations used in this book are from the Holy Bible, New International Version (NIV). Copyright © 1973, 1978, 1984 International Bible Society. Used by permission of Zondervan Bible Publishers. Other Scripture references are from the following sources:

The King James Version of the Bible (KJV).

American Standard Bible (NASB) © 1960, 1962, 1963, 1971, 1973, 1975, and 1977 by the Lockman Foundation, and are used by permission.

Holy Bible, New Living Translation (NLT) (Wheaton, Ill.: Tyndale House Publishers, 1996). Used by permission.

New Revised Standard Version Bible (NRSV). Copyright © 1989 Division of Christian Education of the National Council of the Churches of Christ in the United States of America. Used by permission.

ISBN 0-8499-1691-7

Printed in the United States of America

Contents

Acknowledgments

With gratitude in our hearts we thank God for:

+ Thousands of *Thin Within* participants: whose testimonies affirm the faithfulness of our sovereign God and whose hearts are filled with so much love because of His message of freedom and hope.

+ Our faithful friends who have fervently prayed for us and with us over these many years.

+ Those who have contributed to our personal growth and maturity. Our special thanks to Pastor Ray C. Stedman, from whom we learned about our freedom in Christ, and the pastors at Peninsula Bible Church Brian Morgan, John Hanneman, and Gary Vanderet for their excellent teaching of the inerrant Word of God.

+ Heartfelt gratitude to my dear friend Joy Imboden Overstreet, Co-founder of Thin Within whose contribution will live on through this book and be forever remembered.

+ Roy M. Carlisle, our agent, a faithful servant of God, who has stead-fastly remained at our side through the many challenges of birthing Thin Again and the rebirth of this book.

+ All the people at W Publishing, particularly Mark Sweeney, for their encouragement and forbearance in the publishing of this book.

+ Sally Rackets whose gift of creativity was anointed by God as she crafted our illustrations in record time.

+ High praises to Margaret Copeland for her graciousness and godly patience while she designed and typeset the interior of our book.

+ Pam Sneed who has been a beacon of hope to those who have been seeking God's truth. She has lovingly cared for them through encour-agement and Godly guidance.

+ Bill Dembereckyj and staff, especially Lori Robertson and Lance Hamilton, for capturing the vision and infusing it with their enthusi-asm, zeal, and love for our Lord Jesus Christ.

+ We give high praise to Donna Noell for countless hours at the computer and her infectious good humor in the midst of countless rewrites and revisions of the manuscript and every other project that is placed before her. And to her husband Nelson we are eternally grateful for his faithful troubleshooting.

+ We thank God for Roberta and Ken Eldred, who generously supported us when we needed it the most, and for their steadfast prayers along with those of Dorothy Garcia, Laura Lou Tolles, and Chris Mumford.

+ Sincere thanks to our daughter Amy whose computer expertise and sweet spirit was invaluable in the preparation of this manuscript.

+ Heidi Bylsma—no words can express our admiration and profound respect for your wisdom, insight, enthusiasm, good humor, and seemingly boundless energy in crafting twenty-six years' worth of material into its final form. You truly are a gift from God and we love you.

+ We are eternally grateful to Carney Hawkins whose insight contributed greatly to the development of this material. Her passion and knowledge of the Word of God is greatly to be praised. We thank God for your partnership in setting the captives free.

+ High praise to Diana Johnson, another beloved sister in the Lord who has been a champion for Thin Within and whose heart is dedicated to the truth of God's Word. We are forever indebted to you for your courage to go forth and speak the truth of the Gospel of Christ.

+ Most importantly we give thanks and praise to our Lord, Jesus Christ, who has allowed two very fallible human beings to serve Him. To Him we give all praise, honor, and glory. Our prayer is that more of the captives may be set free to worship, adore, and praise our Sovereign God.

About the Authors

LORD, you establish peace for us;
all that we have accomplished you have done for us.
—Isaiah 26:12

Meet Judy Wardell Halliday, R.N.

My story is one of God's redemption. I praise Him for the way He takes our broken lives and powerfully turns them into His glory. He has healed the brokenness of my life in many ways—including my relationship with my body and with food.

If you are anything like me, you may have discovered the hard way that dieting just doesn't work. I am eternally grateful for the joy, peace, and contentment I now have where food, weight, and my body are concerned, but it has not always been so. As with all treasures worth possessing, the abundant life I now savor has come after many years of searching, much like the Israelites looking for the promised land. What could have been a short trip took me some forty years of wandering in the wilderness. I pray that God will use my prolonged travels to make your path much shorter!

For most of my teenage years, weight was not an issue. But at age twenty, due to a series of traumatic events, I took a downward spiral. I gained thirty-eight pounds and was bingeing and purging several times a day, which created a cycle of shame and self-abuse. You will see my story woven throughout the pages of this book. Although the particulars of our lives may differ, you may find that we have shared a similar path. Our great God can take the things that we find utterly hopeless and use them for His glory. He did just that, by using my struggles with my weight and the subsequent despondency to propel me into a quest, searching for answers to some of the basic questions of life: What is the purpose for my life? Why am I here?

Ultimately, many years later, I was lead to the cross of Christ—but being a slow learner, I took the circuitous route. I studied all sorts of religions, both old and "new," from Eastern religions to New Age, astrology to E-meters, rebirthing to Rolfing. I was looking for anything that might answer my probing questions.

Energized by my search for meaning, I managed to prop myself up with "positive thinking." Eventually I stopped bingeing and purging and lost the excess weight.

When I became a registered nurse, I found myself drawn to psychiatry. I loved connecting with people who were considered out of society's mainstream. As I spoke to their hearts, I often found them experiencing unexpected moments of lucidity. Sharing those moments was a true gift, and I remember them as special times of my life. While practicing nursing at night, I practiced modern dance by day, and ultimately joined a professional dance company. I appeared to have it all together, but inside, my soul was still searching.

In 1975, I met Joy Imboden Overstreet, a fellow struggler, who had begun observing the behavior of naturally thin people—those who never *diet*, but who remain thin from within. As a result of this study Thin Within workshops evolved. Together we were astonished at the success of people losing weight, and keeping it off.

In 1985, *Thin Within*, the book was published, and Thin Within, the organization, flourished. But in the process, Thin Within became my identity. It was my family and my passion, which I served seven days a week. Thin Within had become my god. I deified it just as I had deified food and exercise. I was without a weight problem, but I was not really free. I had simply exchanged addictions!

At this time, a friend asked me to go to church—something that was definitely not a priority in my life. Out of curiosity I went, and was interested to hear about a personal relationship with Christ. I saw married couples who had something that I longed for—an intimacy, a warmth, a love for which I yearned. Afraid of making a mistake in a relationship, I had always shied away from marriage. Nevertheless, it was something I'd always wanted. I now recognize that God was using this area of my life to "tenderize" me and speak to my heart.

My friend then introduced me to the Bible. It's embarrassing, but that was the last place I wanted to look for answers to the basic questions of life. I wanted to find the answers in something new and revolutionary, not in something two thousand years old. But as I read, I was stunned that the

Bible had a blueprint not only for marriage, but for my life. Finally I had hope! My hungry heart led me to read on and to see God's plan for dealing properly with our bodies and food. I was astounded to learn that the *body is designed to be a temple of God* (1 Corinthians 3:16).

Then, as if to nudge my wavering hand, a financial crisis hit. Suddenly Thin Within was facing bankruptcy. The world into which I had poured my blood, sweat, and tears came crashing down around me. I was devastated. The life I had carefully constructed was in shambles, and there was no place to turn except up. In His mercy, God met me where I was, and I asked Jesus Christ to be my Lord and Savior.

Psalm 127:1 says, *Unless the LORD builds the house, they labor in vain who build it.*

God salvaged a remnant and began rebuilding the "house" of Thin Within based on a biblical foundation. He gave me a ravenous appetite for His word. I learned that much of what we were teaching in Thin Within was aligned with the Bible (that was thrilling), but some was not (that was embarrassing). He also showed me that my performance had nothing to do with my identity; it was about Him giving me a new heart.

As if that were not enough, God answered my fervent prayer and hand-picked for me the most wonderful man in the world, to whom I have been married since 1984. Together we have had the privilege of serving God and seeing Him transform thousands of minds, hearts, and bodies through Thin Within workshops. We are thankful that you, dear reader, have chosen to join us on this exciting journey.

Meet Arthur Halliday, M.D.

The first forty years of my life were pretty unremarkable: typical upbringing in a small Kansas town, left home and church at seventeen, physics degree from college, challenging job with the Atomic Energy Commission, career change, medical degree at twenty-seven, marriage, three wonderful children, very rewarding professional career practicing medicine with my two brothers, and a house overlooking the country club. Then, because my priorities were primarily worldly, my life began a ten-year slide that ended in a pile of rubble, with two failed marriages, a mountain of debt, and three children who wondered—as I did—what was wrong with their dad. I started reading self-help books, going to seminars, and talking to people, as I tried to figure out what was wrong. For the first time, I began to look inward and I became aware of a cavernous void deep within.

In the fall of 1981, a new disease was reported in a group of previously healthy young men in Los Angeles. It quickly became the worst pandemic in history—AIDS. As the disease spread, I volunteered to work in an AIDS clinic in San Francisco and saw my life change radically over the next six years as I watched hundreds of young men and women die horrible deaths.

It was during this challenging time that I met Judy and began to get to know her and her Christian friends, many of whom began praying for me. I started going to church with her as well as reading the Bible and praying. What happened next changed my life forever. God allowed me to see a visible, tangible portrayal of the yearning of my own heart when I spoke with one of my dying AIDS patients. He was a very bright, well-educated admissions officer at a local college. As he confided in me regarding his promiscuity, I was amazed that he would have engaged in such risky behavior, knowing what was at stake. I asked him why.

"Dr. Halliday," he said, "I was looking for love." I was stunned. There I was—the scientifically oriented, well-trained doctor, watching him die because he had tried to find the love that all of us seek. And I didn't have a clue as to what to say or do to try to help him. I realized then that he was a portrait of myself—longing, thirsty, empty, his soul a cavernous spiritual wasteland. He died just a short time after our talk, never experiencing the love he so desperately sought.

About two weeks later, on June 25, 1984, I was awakened during the night and experienced what could only have been the presence and power of God. I tasted the depth, height, and length of love that knows no measure—and I gave my life to Him.

I discovered that God loves us and accepts us as we are and where we are right now. He will gladly enter the life that is surrendered. He doesn't wait for us to get it all together first. It is our prayer that you will rest more deeply in this fact of God's never-ending love and unconditional acceptance as a result of spending thirty days with us in the pages of this book.

God truly is the answer that so many of us seek elsewhere. His desire is to meet you and overwhelm you with His love poured forth on your life. Thank you for joining us on this exciting journey.

Introduction

Listen, listen to me, and eat what is good,
and your soul will delight in the richest of fare.
Give ear and come to me; hear me, that your soul may live.
I will make an everlasting covenant with you,
my faithful love promised to David.
—Isaiah 55:2–3

God's amazing grace abounds between the covers of this book. Here you will find provocative and inspiring testimonies as well as a vast resource of effective exercises and tools with which to pave a God-honoring path. As you journey on this path to peace and freedom with food, eating, and your body, you will find information that will stimulate, enlighten, and encourage you. Most of all, you will experience an invitation whispered to your soul from God—an invitation to enter in, to draw nearer, to plunge deeper, to experience more fully the joy and abundant living that He intends for you.

If you wonder how we can make such promises, Matthew 19:26 says it all: *"With man this is impossible, but with God all things are possible!"* God rejoices in His involvement in our lives. He promises that He has a plan, a hope, and a future for each of us (Jeremiah 29:11). As you dare to dream big dreams with us, over the next thirty days you will see that God is sufficient and satisfying and that His love and grace is grander than anything you can imagine.

It is no accident that this book is in your hands right now. God's desire is that you would hear His voice whispering to you as you read the words written on these pages.

The material in the book is based on a foundation of four cornerstones:

1. It is aligned with the word of God and is based on God's amazing grace.
2. It works—thousands of graduates have reached and maintained their natural size since 1975.

3. It is medically sound—no bizarre diets or forbidden foods—with results of improved physical, emotional, and spiritual health.

4. It provides a path that will lead you to a godly perspective of your body as well as to the abundant life.

We have included "Medical Moments" to give you confirmation and insights as to various physiological components of this program, how it works and how well your body will respond to it and why.

We know how hard it can be to unlearn many things we have come to depend on over the years, even if they haven't worked. However, you can rejoice because you will see results starting on Day One. Throughout *Thin Within* you will use the "Observation and Correction" tool. This is a tool that will allow you to take note of your current behavior from a nonjudgmental position and make corrections accordingly. As you walk in the transforming power of God's grace you will have the freedom to do so without self condemnation.

We are thankful for the transformation that has taken place both with Thin Within and in our personal lives by the power of Almighty God. He has revealed to us over many years that He is in control of life and His dreams are far greater than our own. His plans are to give us a future and a hope that stretches the length of eternity.

Our prayer is that each of you will see more clearly that God loves and accepts you completely. His desire is to transform each of us from within. His plans are wondrous beyond fathoming.

During the next thirty days you will not count a single calorie or fat gram. In fact, you will be encouraged to throw out any and all the dieting foods or paraphernalia you may have. Sound radical? We agree. But unless you love fat-free blue cheese salad dressing you will love getting rid of it to make room for the real thing! You will learn that you can be the size God designed you to be while eating the foods you enjoy. You will also learn how to make food choices based not only on what tastes good but what is excellent in the eyes of God.

Do you know any naturally thin people who eat only diet foods? Neither do we! You will learn to eat as a naturally thin person and become thin—from within. Will you become thin on the outside, too? Absolutely! The wonderful thing is that as you become thin from within, you will remain that way for the rest of your life. Will you starve while on this program? No! You are welcome to eat what you enjoy whenever you are *truly* hungry.

You will put away your "club of condemnation" and, instead, learn to walk in newness of a grace-filled life in the present moment. Together we will feast on the sustenance of God who has promised to be so incredibly satisfying! You will *taste and see that the* LORD *is good* (Psalm 34:8).

Many of us have run to seminars, classes, self-help books, drugs, promiscuity, and, yes, even to food, to fill the emptiness in our heart that only He can satisfy. God desires to meet you and overwhelm you with His love poured forth on your life, heart, and soul.

During the next thirty days our focus won't be only on externals or appearances. Our purpose is to outline for you a program whose goal is your optimum health—initially your physical health, but ultimately your emotional and spiritual health as well. Our hope and prayer is that you will journey with us and realize a truly restored temple of the Holy Spirit and a life that reflects God's glory.

As you will see, Thin Within is very different from diets!

Are you ready to be set free . . .

+ from the compelling call of food? (Galatians 5:1)
+ from reacting to the demands of your impulses that say, "I want it and I want it now"? (Micah 6:8)
+ from past failures? (1 Kings 2:4)

Are you ready . . .

+ to respond to the high calling of a God who loves you and longs to secure you in His sovereignty? (Isaiah 25:8)
+ to live the abundant life? *Christ in you, the hope of glory* (Colossians 1:27).

Are you with us? There is one who is the master travel guide, so let's follow Him!

Dear God,

Thank You for being with me as I begin this journey. I must admit I am a bit hesitant about this process because I have "started" and "stopped" so many times before. I pray that I might see You as never before and be set free from my heartaches over food, eating, and my body. Lord, I know diets or other things I have tried have not worked in the long run. I know You have something so much better for me, so I invite You to show me truth. Open my eyes and release me from the chains that bind me. Open my heart unto You! In Jesus' name, Amen.

Before You Begin

Blessed are those whose strength is in you,
who have set their hearts on pilgrimage.
As they pass through the Valley of Baca,
they make it a place of springs;
the autumn rains also cover it with pools.
They go from strength to strength,
till each appears before God in Zion.
—Psalm 84:5–7

A promising new road beckons, inviting you on a journey to freedom—freedom from concerns about food, eating, and your body. A great adventure awaits where you will discover much about yourself and the one who created you. God will be your guide on this journey, and He is present and waiting to accompany you. The empowerment of His Holy Spirit is already active and at work.

Before we get underway, let's look at where you have been and where you are today. To do that, we've provided the following questionnaire—"Where I've Come From." On Day Twenty-Nine you will complete this questionnaire again and compare it with the one you finish today. By that time you will find yourself far from where you are today. We are sure the results will astound you. God is an awesome God. Expect great things from our mighty Lord. He won't disappoint you.

Where I've Come From
Brief History

1. How was your weight as a child? (under 12 years old):

    Underweight   Ideal Weight   Somewhat Overweight   Very overweight

2. How old were you when you first decided you had a weight problem?

    | 1–7 years | 13–19 | 30–39 | 50–59 |
    | 8–12 | 20–29 | 40–49 | over 60 |

3. How frequently do you weigh yourself?

Once a day   2–5 times a week   2–5 times a month   Very rarely

4. How was your father's weight when you were young?

Underweight   Ideal weight   Somewhat overweight   Very overweight

5. How was your mother's weight when you were young?

Underweight   Ideal weight   Somewhat overweight   Very overweight

On the following questions, circle the number that best applies:

6. How much of the time are you on a diet or sacrificing certain types of foods?

1	2	3	4	5	6	7	8	9	10
Always									Never

7. How frequently do you eat foods you really enjoy?

1	2	3	4	5	6	7	8	9	10
Always									Never

8. How often do you think of yourself as a thin person?

1	2	3	4	5	6	7	8	9	10
Always									Never

9. Can you visualize or imagine yourself at your natural size—the size God designed you to be?

1	2	3	4	5	6	7	8	9	10
Always									Never

10. Do you think you are aware of your body's hunger and fullness signals?

1	2	3	4	5	6	7	8	9	10
Always									Never

Imagine that you had a fuel gauge for your stomach, much like that on a car, which registered how empty or full you were:

11. At what point on the gauge do you usually start eating?

0	1	2	3	4	5	6	7	8	9	10
Empty					Comfy					Stuffed

12. At what point on the gauge do you usually stop eating?

0	1	2	3	4	5	6	7	8	9	10
Empty					Comfy					Stuffed

What are your current concerns? Rate each item listed below.

13. Spending too much time worrying about my weight or eating behavior

0	1	2	3	4	5	6	7	8	9	10

Serious Problem   No Problem

14. Weighing frequently

0	1	2	3	4	5	6	7	8	9	10

Serious Problem   No Problem

15. Anorexia Nervosa

0	1	2	3	4	5	6	7	8	9	10

Serious Problem   No Problem

16. Bulimia

0	1	2	3	4	5	6	7	8	9	10

Serious Problem   No Problem

17. Disliking my body

0	1	2	3	4	5	6	7	8	9	10

Serious Problem   No Problem

18. Thinking too much about food

0	1	2	3	4	5	6	7	8	9	10

Serious Problem   No Problem

19. Snacking (between meals or at night)

0	1	2	3	4	5	6	7	8	9	10

Serious Problem   No Problem

20. Alcoholic beverages

0	1	2	3	4	5	6	7	8	9	10

Serious Problem   No Problem

21. Cigarettes

0	1	2	3	4	5	6	7	8	9	10

Serious Problem   No Problem

22. Feeling guilty about what I eat

0	1	2	3	4	5	6	7	8	9	10

Serious Problem   No Problem

23. Not caring at all about what I eat

0	1	2	3	4	5	6	7	8	9	10

Serious Problem   No Problem

24. Eating out of stress or boredom

| 0 | 1 | 2 | 3 | 4 | 5 | 6 | 7 | 8 | 9 | 10 |
Serious Problem | | | | | | | | | No Problem

25. Social eating (parties, restaurants)

| 0 | 1 | 2 | 3 | 4 | 5 | 6 | 7 | 8 | 9 | 10 |
Serious Problem | | | | | | | | | No Problem

In general, how do you rate your life in the following areas?

26. Health

| 1 | 2 | 3 | 4 | 5 | 6 | 7 | 8 | 9 | 10 |
Poor | | | | | | | | | Excellent

27. Energy level

| 0 | 1 | 2 | 3 | 4 | 5 | 6 | 7 | 8 | 9 | 10 |
Low | | | | | | | | | High

28. Physical activity

| 0 | 1 | 2 | 3 | 4 | 5 | 6 | 7 | 8 | 9 | 10 |
Sedentary | | | | | | | | | Extremely Active

29. Productivity

| 0 | 1 | 2 | 3 | 4 | 5 | 6 | 7 | 8 | 9 | 10 |
Low | | | | | | | | | High

30. Job satisfaction (consider student or housewife as a job)

| 0 | 1 | 2 | 3 | 4 | 5 | 6 | 7 | 8 | 9 | 10 |
Unsatisfying | | | | | | | | | Very Satisfying

31. Close relationships (friends)

| 0 | 1 | 2 | 3 | 4 | 5 | 6 | 7 | 8 | 9 | 10 |
Unsatisfying | | | | | | | | | Very Satisfying

32. Family relationships

| 0 | 1 | 2 | 3 | 4 | 5 | 6 | 7 | 8 | 9 | 10 |
Unsatisfying | | | | | | | | | Very Satisfying

33. Sex life

| 0 | 1 | 2 | 3 | 4 | 5 | 6 | 7 | 8 | 9 | 10 |
Unsatisfying | | | | | | | | | Very Satisfying

34. Ability to speak up for what I want

| 0 | 1 | 2 | 3 | 4 | 5 | 6 | 7 | 8 | 9 | 10 |
Difficult | | | | | | | | | Easy

35. Level of self-esteem

0	1	2	3	4	5	6	7	8	9	10
Low										High

Thank you for taking the time to complete the questionnaire. It will be beneficial to reflect back on your answers on Day Twenty-Nine.

Blessed are you for setting your heart on a pilgrimage! As we pass through valleys, deserts, and forests, our God will be our strength and our guide.

So get your walking shoes on. We're on our way.

Prayer

Dear God, as I look back over where I've been and where I am today, I'm humbled and hungry for a way out of my dilemma. I find myself in need of Your grace, Your mercy, Your tenderness, and Your compassion. Thank You for offering that and so much more. I must admit that I feel a little reticent about what lies ahead. Yet I am thankful that You journey with me as I embark on this quest to become more fully what You have created me to be. In Jesus' name I pray, Amen.

Part I
Experiencing the Refreshment of Freedom

∽

Free to Enjoy God's Lavish Love

The LORD your God is with you,
he is mighty to save.
He will take great delight in you,
he will quiet you with his love,
he will rejoice over you with singing.
—Zephaniah 3:17

Welcome to an enlightening personal journey that will direct you on a path to peace and freedom. On this road you will have the delight of discovering the plan and purpose that God has especially for you. He has designed this plan for your benefit, to give you a future and a hope (Jeremiah 29:11).

No matter where you have been or how you have fared, we rejoice that God has allowed our paths to merge for the next thirty days. Our mighty Way Maker will direct our steps as we continue down this path of discovery and adventure. During this time you will find yourself drawn closer to God, the lover of your soul and the designer of your body, the one who purchased your liberty. He longs for you to see His handiwork displayed in a most miraculous masterpiece—*you.*

He wants to impress deeply into the soft clay of your heart His unfathomable love for you. This love is not based on your performance. It is not based on whether you are thin, thick, tall, short, or whether or not you "succeed" at applying the Thin Within principles that we will share with you.

As Amy, one of our graduates, writes, "Thin Within changed my life in so many positive ways. Since it is based on the word of God, it involved love and acceptance. I learned that it is God who could transform me into the person I longed to be."

But food does not bring us near to God; we are no worse if we do not eat, and no better if we do (1 Corinthians 8:8).

No matter whether you eat or don't eat, the simple fact is God is crazy about you. Whether you are ten pounds or a hundred and ten pounds overweight, God loves you exactly the way you are. There is absolutely nothing you can do to make Him love you more or less now than a moment ago or a year ago. *Jesus Christ is the same yesterday and today and forever* (Hebrews 13:8). If a quest for the "perfect" body has led you to try diet upon diet, you may have had some temporary results, but not without a price. Dieting ultimately leads to a heavy heart. The truth is that while diets and dieting rules may seem like the answer, they have a ninety-five percent failure rate. However, now it is time to be renewed in your belief that God is able and willing to lead you to freedom from food rules and to the abundant life!

Ruth shares, "I lost over one hundred pounds with a popular weight-loss program. But I never dealt with why I had an eating problem in the first place. As a result, losing the weight was more like a Band-aid and I quickly regained over fifty pounds. I love Thin Within because it helped me to see what is at the heart of my struggles with eating. It encouraged me to invite God into the process and to welcome His touch of healing. I've now lost over twenty of the pounds I had gained back, but even more, my heart is being healed as well."

The struggle with the dieting treadmill is made more difficult by the fact that we long for the flavor of authentic blue cheese dressing and settle resentfully for a fat-free variety instead. We crave Häagen-Dazs ice cream and instead tolerate low-fat frozen yogurt. While utilizing artificial sweeteners and artificial fats, we aren't enjoying our food and, too often, we aren't enjoying our lives either, even if our bodies get smaller for a season. In short, when we are dieting we never get that chance to be who we really are.

Susan dropped sixty pounds using the Thin Within Keys to Conscious Eating, which we will describe to you in a moment. "Before the workshop, I had tried hypnosis and many expensive weight-loss systems. But if you tell me I can't eat chocolate cake, I'll want it every day. I didn't do well on diets with rigid restrictions. With Thin Within I can live a normal lifestyle."

Thin Within is not a diet plan. It is a way of life. If you prayerfully apply yourself to what we share in these pages, you will discover that you can be the person God made you to be, perfectly aligning your preference for chocolate fudge and pecan pie with your natural God-given size. It is a process that requires time and commitment. However, it is also full of enriching self-discovery. As you choose to use the tools in this book, you will be amazed at the changes you will see in your body and heart in just thirty days.

There is nothing more refreshing than authentic living. God wants this for you. He created you to be unique. As you begin to live authentically, you will discover the abundant life Jesus talked about—a life that is deeply satisfying. When you allow the Lord to meet your needs, you will find a fulfillment that you never knew existed. You will begin to need less food as you realize that much of your eating has been triggered by something that food really can't satisfy. You will begin to see that you can become authentically *thin within*, from your heart and soul outward. This external change will reflect the miracle that is taking place in a heart set free.

As you release yourself into God's capable hands, as you release your hesitation to trust your body's signals, as you release your "heart hunger" (which we will discuss later), you will find that you release weight as well. In Thin Within, we don't use the term "lose weight." To lose something usually means we hope to find it again. Instead we talk about "releasing" weight.

While working through these pages, rest assured that you will never be condemned for making mistakes. Instead we will encourage you with each mistake or shortcoming to seek the Lord. You will be asked to take note of your missteps and make adjustments. That's it. At Thin Within, we call that "observation and correction." We promise never to wag a finger at you. Thin Within is a grace-based approach to food and weight management.

In the spirit of grace, a word of caution is appropriate at this point. Please don't turn any of what we share here into a set of laws that you must keep to be "good" or to please God. We want you to be liberated from the bondage of diets and to experience joy, peace, and freedom. As Bob, one of our participants, said, "One of the things I like about the tools and the entire Thin Within approach is that I can choose to use the charts and graphs if I need to. Other times, when I am living more naturally according to this way of life, I find I don't consciously need to use the tools. Either way, there is flexibility and a sense of freedom."

We are all too familiar with food rules and laws. It seems that every diet has its list of dos and don'ts. "Is this one thirty percent fat or is it ten percent fat? What foods are 'legal' for protein sources? How many grams of protein are in two ounces of cheese?" On and on it goes until our heads spin. God speaks directly to this dieting merry-go-round in the Bible.

Since you died with Christ to the basic principles of this world, why, as though you still belonged to it, do you submit to its rules: "Do not handle! Do not taste! Do not touch!"? These are all destined to perish with use, because they are based on human commands and teachings. Such regulations indeed have an appearance of wisdom, with their self-imposed worship, their false humility and their harsh treatment of the body, but they lack any value in restraining sensual indulgence (Colossians 2:20–23).

We are blessedly free from all of that worry and concern. "Before I came to Thin Within," says Julia, "I was a part of a program that impressed on me that if I love God enough I will eat between the parameters of hunger and fullness. Somehow for me this simple principle got turned into a *law* and a *rule*. I found myself more than ever focused on food and on my sin. With this grace-oriented approach, I found that heeding the voice of the Spirit of God took my focus away from food and eating rules. I have gotten to know the body that God has given me and I have, without self-condemnation, identified what 'empty' and 'comfortable' feel like."

My Current Relationship with Food

Before we share the keys to conscious eating, let's look first at how you relate to food and eating. Imagine yourself at the movies. Picture in your mind a movie in full color and surround sound, starring you. You are eating the last meal you had before you opened this book today. Maybe it was this morning's breakfast, maybe it was last night's dinner. Envision yourself on the theater screen eating that meal.

Where are you?

What is going on in the environment?

Is it noisy and distracting? Or quiet and serene?

Are you seated at a table set up for eating?

Do you notice what you are eating?

Are you concentrating on your food? Or are you busy talking?

Are you thinking about other things while you are eating?

Are you reading, watching TV, or doing something else?

Were you truly hungry when you began eating?

Were you eating for other reasons?

Was it just "time" to eat?

Observe yourself eating the food. Notice how fast or slow you were eating.

Do you ever have an empty mouth or put your fork down while eating?

Do you taste each bite?

Do you enjoy each item?

Is each item what you really wanted?

Do you wash the food down with liquids?

Now, notice your emotional state.

Are you attempting to swallow some unexpressed emotions along with your food?

Did you clean your plate?

Was there a time during this meal that you noticed you felt satisfied but continued eating anyway?

After you were finished eating, did you nibble at the food left on your plate or on other people's plates?

Did you overeat?

How did you feel at the end of the meal? Satisfied? Stuffed?

Did you feel guilty?

Were you aware of the entire meal experience?

Was this meal a pleasant or an unpleasant experience for you? What made it that way?

Now the movie of your meal is ending. Once the curtains close, write in the space provided below what your thoughts, impressions, and insights were during your viewing of your movie.

1. How did you relate to the food?
2. What were your emotions and feelings?
3. What is your overall assessment of the experience?

I ate because I wanted to try the green chile Jenny had sent me. But also because Skip was hungry.

At Thin Within we use the observation and correction tool to lead you in the direction of your God-given weight goal, which includes being at peace with food and with your body. What you have just done in the activity above is *observation*. When we change behaviors from things that don't work to things that do, we call that the *correction* part of the equation. And observation and correction are what the keys to conscious eating are designed to help you do. After thirty days, when you reread what you have written above, you will probably be amazed at how much observing and correcting you have actually done.

About the Keys to Conscious Eating

In the pages that follow, we will share principles that will enable you to be at peace with food, your body, and others around you. These are not dieting *laws*; instead they are "keys" that can lead to a better life. We believe that these keys to conscious eating will unlock the ability that God placed inside of you—the power to participate in your own transformation from the inside out.

I pray also that the eyes of your heart may be enlightened in order that you may know the hope to which he has called you, the riches of his glorious inheritance in the saints, and his incomparably great power for us who believe. That power is like the working of his mighty strength (Ephesians 1:18–19).

Keys to Conscious Eating

1. Eat only when my body is hungry. This principle is at the heart of becoming aware of your body and what it needs. Most of us actually eat much more food than our bodies require in order to function efficiently. Consider for a moment how often during the past few days you have allowed your body to feel hungry. This week begin to listen to the God-given cue of "hunger" and respond accordingly. This probably sounds obvious to you. The fact is much of our overeating occurs when we aren't really hungry, so if you can't figure our whether you are hungry or not, give your body the benefit of the doubt. "When in doubt, leave it out." (Don't eat.) *I am the* LORD *your God, . . . Open wide your mouth and I will fill it* (Psalm 81:10).

2. Reduce the number of distractions in order to eat in a calm environment. There is a delightful experience that awaits you at each meal. However, if you are like most of us, your mealtimes are often chaotic instead of calm. A chaotic environment produces chaotic eating. Ponder relishing a quiet meal, where you can *be still, and know that [He is] God* (Psalm 46:10) when you eat. You will discover that eating really can be a more satisfying experience. Allow yourself the pleasure of being focused on your food. At Thin Within, we call this eating in "present time." If your mind is elsewhere or if you are distracted, you are less likely to enjoy your food. You will also find yourself going back for "seconds" because you were not fully present the first time around. The Lord wants us to experience both His provisions and His peace. Mealtimes can be an opportunity to turn off the TV or disruptive music, and put aside your reading. In the process, we can then praise Him for the sight, the smell, and the taste of each bite of food.

3. Eat when sitting down. Americans are famous for eating on the run, and much of our unconscious or mindless eating is done while driving. If you eat on the run or while standing at the kitchen counter, you aren't fully focused on the food or enjoying present-time eating. When this happens, you may hear yourself saying, "I haven't had a thing to eat all day."

We will encourage you throughout these thirty days to remain in the present moment and to relish it for the pleasure it brings. If you sit down and take time to focus on giving your body the fuel it needs, your mind will record the fact that you have eaten. Often, in our hurry-on-the-go lifestyles, we charge ahead and our hearts and minds feel as if they haven't been refreshed. [And then he said,] *"Refresh yourself with something to eat; then you can go." So the two of them sat down to eat and drink together* (Judges 19:5–6).

4. Eat when my body and mind are relaxed. Take a quiet moment to invite the Lord of the wind and waves into your meal. The one who said, "Peace, be still" is eager for you to enjoy freedom from anxiety at your mealtimes. God wants to free you from worry and to infuse your life with peace. *Do not be anxious for your life, as to what you shall eat, or what you shall drink. . . . Is not life more than food, and the body more important than clothing? . . . Seek first His kingdom, and His righteousness; and all these things shall be added to you* (Matthew 6:25, 33, NASB).

5. Eat and drink the food and beverages my body enjoys. Relish this as the opportunity to be authentic. With a thankful spirit and no guilt whatsoever, you can eat and enjoy whatever your heart desires and whatever your body calls for. You are free to be real with yourself and with God. You will discover how trustworthy your body is as you melt down to the size God created you to be. *"Can't you see that what you eat won't defile you? Food doesn't come in contact with your heart, but only passes through the stomach and then comes out again." (By saying this, he showed that every kind of food is acceptable.)* (Mark 7:18–19, NLT)

Too often, we get caught up in thinking we are "good" or "bad" based on what we eat. Food can't cleanse the heart no matter how little fat or how much fiber it contains. Be liberated and rejoice as you rid yourself of such thoughts and other dieting rules. *For the kingdom of God is not a matter of eating and drinking, but of righteousness, peace and joy in the Holy Spirit* (Romans 14:17).

There are no forbidden foods. If you have food allergies or a medical condition that would require abstinence from certain foods, by all means heed your doctor's recommendations. But aside from that, enjoy God's wonderful provisions. We might, however, be tempted to take this to an extreme, to abuse or misuse food. It's important for us to remember that *"Everything is permissible for me"—but not everything is beneficial. "Everything is permissible for me"—but I will not be mastered by anything* (1 Corinthians 6:12). When unsure, ask God what your body needs in order to feel and operate at its best. You will then know what will be an appropriate choice.

6. Pay attention to my food while eating. During many of your meals you will dine with others. We are enriched both by our interaction with others and by the nourishment and delight provided by the food we eat. We experience maximum satisfaction as we give our full attention to each in turn. How can you apply this key? We suggest that you attempt to establish a rhythm as you eat. Look at your food, take a bite, chew deliberately, and fully experience the flavor. Then set your fork down and focus on your companions, giving them your full attention. Return to focus on your food, and continue this back-and-forth process. As you practice this rhythm you will be able to do this without giving it much thought. Your meals will be more intentional and more enjoyable.

7. Eat slowly and savor each bite. People often eat when they are distracted or distressed. Since we are not eating consciously at these times, the result can be overindulgence. If we eat only when we are hungry, and if we sit down, relax, and focus on our food, we will truly enjoy the eating experience and we can stop the habitual "inhaling" of food. You can enjoy your food, one small bite at a time. *Go and enjoy choice food and sweet drinks* (Nehemiah 8:10). As you "enjoy choice food and sweet drinks," you will be surprised how little food it takes to make you feel satisfied. As you eat more slowly, your stomach can accurately signal your brain as to when your physical need for food has been satisfied.

8. Stop *before* my body is "full." In other words, stop at a place of comfort before your body is "full" or "stuffed." Many participants find this problematic to apply. They may develop an awareness of what physical hunger feels like, but then, once they begin to eat, they roll right on past the appropriate stopping point. Twenty minutes later, they are surprised to find themselves needing to unbutton their pants or become horizontal in order to be "comfortable." However, once they take the time to slow down and to savor their food, stopping at a place of comfort isn't quite as challenging. If you feel "full," or "stuffed" when you stop eating, your stomach is being stretched and you have actually eaten more than your body needs. If you are tempted to eat beyond a "comfortable" point, remind yourself that no temptation is beyond His reach. *God is faithful; he will not let you be tempted beyond what you can bear. But when you are tempted, he will also provide a way out so that you can stand up under it* (1 Corinthians 10:13).

Again, please do not allow these keys to become "rules." They are meant only to be tools to serve you. For the next thirty days we encourage you to give these tools a test run. We include record sheets where you can, if you choose, keep track of various aspects of your journey. With that in mind, feel free to write in this book, make notes, use any assignments that may assist you in applying godly principles.

Commit yourself to spending a few minutes each day sitting quietly in the presence of God, asking for His wisdom. Then read *Thin Within* and absorb the concepts presented. Refer to your Bible when a verse is referenced. You may even want to have a journal to chronicle your progress. The more you look to God and are open to His leading on this journey, the more likely you are to experience the abundant life that has been given to us in Christ.

Take Action

+ Experience hunger before eating. This is key #1 and it will help you to get started on your path to freedom.
+ On your first day in the program, we ask that you make a commitment to dispose of dieting paraphernalia. Whether you have been stuck on the dieting treadmill, despaired of diets long ago, or have never dieted, please write your commitment below. You might write something like this: Today I refuse any longer to eat with my eye on labels or according to food laws of any kind. I will not weigh and measure my food any longer. I will apply the keys to conscious eating for the next thirty days.

_____

_____

_____

Now is the time to throw out every diet book, calorie counter, magazine article, and diet product you have collected. If you are currently using diet pills, shots, or liquid protein, we ask that you consult your physician. If you obtain his or her blessing, toss them into the trash while repeating your commitment out loud.

Jeremiah 29:11 says, *"For I know the plans I have for you,"* declares the LORD, *"plans to prosper you and not to harm you, plans to give you hope and a future."*

✦ Acknowledge that you believe what Jeremiah 29:11 says by personalizing this verse in a written prayer. Here is an example of what we mean:

I believe, Lord, that you have plans for me. I believe Your plans are not to harm me, but to give me a hope and a future, Lord. I thank You that your plan isn't a diet but a way of life in which I am no longer anxious about food, where I can begin to trust the body You have designed for me. I put my trust in You and will follow the leading of the Spirit within. I choose to believe You, Lord. Amen.

Now it's your turn!

_____

_____

Your Success Story

✦ In the following space, please jot down any new insights God has revealed to you while reading today. Journaling daily will help you become aware of your path toward conscious eating and your natural God-given size.

_____

_____

_____

✦ Whether you are confident or skeptical as you journey with us for the next thirty days, we invite you to experience God's love, which He offers freely to you. While it costs you nothing, it cost Him a great deal. Why did he pay it? Because you are worth it. You are His treasure.

Verses to Ponder

Therefore do not worry, saying, "What will we eat?" or "What will we drink?" or "What will we wear?" (Matthew 6:31, NRSV)

I have loved you with an everlasting love; I have drawn you with loving-kindness. I will build you up again and you will be rebuilt. . . . Again you will take up your tambourines and go out to dance with the joyful (Jeremiah 31:3–4).

Prayer

Dear Lord, thank You that You have a plan for me that includes a hope and a future. I want to discover what those plans are. I have struggled with food and eating and my body for so many years. Lord, help me to follow You as I long for the changes You will work deep within me. I trust that this is the way You have chosen for me for the remainder of my life. In Jesus' name, Amen.

Medical Moment

Many people wonder about the validity of an approach that considers all foods "legal" in a program designed to help them lose weight. We are so used to structured diets and food programs that require us to follow food laws. However, we have discovered that as people eat with freedom they tend to make wiser and healthier food choices. When people strive to adhere to a strict diet, most often they deny themselves what they most desire. This results in an even stronger attraction to the "forbidden" food. As we encourage people to set aside dieting laws and rules and to enjoy whatever God has made as their body calls for it, they eat smaller amounts of foods that have even been considered "off limits." They seem to flourish and release excess weight, knowing that they will be able to enjoy this newly found freedom for the rest of their lives.

—ARTHUR HALLIDAY, M.D.

Success Tools

+ Eat when you are hungry. Begin to notice all the different occasions when you think about eating. Take stock of those times and wait for your stomach to tell you it's empty.
+ Use the Observations and Corrections Chart below as often as you like during your thirty-day journey. Use it to observe which Thin Within keys to conscious eating you're using and which ones you're not using. When you eat or drink, place a check mark or star beside the key

that you used. If there are empty boxes at the end of the day, that will be an indication for you to pay more attention to that particular key.

✦ Have fun with this chart. Personalize it if you want, drawing lines between each of your eating occasions. Do whatever best suits you— use gold stars, stickers, or colored pens, knowing that every time you make your special mark you're a step farther down that road toward becoming authentically *thin within*. As you progress you will notice those keys you have diligently applied. Those that don't have your special mark beside them will require prayerful attention and application in order to continue to progress. For example, after three days you observe that you only sat down to eat twice and that was in the car. Due to that observation you are now ready to correct and eat more consciously by sitting down while eating.

Thin Within Observations and Corrections Chart—Day 1

Observations	Day 1
1. I ate when my body was hungry.	
2. I ate in a calm environment by reducing distractions.	
3. I ate when I was sitting.	
4. I ate when my body and mind were relaxed.	
5. I ate and drank the things my body enjoyed.	
6. I paid attention to my food while eating.	
7. I ate slowly, savoring each bite.	
8. I stopped before my body was full.	

Thin Within Wisdom

It's not *what* you eat; it's *when* you eat *and* how much.

Getting to Know the Me God Has Made

Even to your old age and gray hairs I am he,
I am he who will sustain you.
I have made you and I will carry you;
I will sustain you and I will rescue you.
—Isaiah 46:4

God ordained that you would walk the earth at this point in history—that you would love, live, and experience all the wonders and challenges that life offers. Nothing about your life was, is, or will ever be hidden from His sight. He is the one who guides, sustains, carries, and rescues you. None of your days is without purpose. It is our prayer that, as we begin the second day of our travels together, you will find yourself depending more deeply on the Lord and that you will learn much as you walk beside the one who created the starry host and the vast oceans. He desires you to know Him—to be in relationship with Him, and to be absolutely authentic before Him.

My Relationship with Myself and My Relationship with God

In these first miles of our journey, your quest will lead you through many interesting discoveries, not the least of which will be insights into yourself and into the God who created you. We will discuss beliefs and how they may affect you on your journey. Because many changes are in store for you, you will find it helpful to have a record that reflects where you began at the onset of our sojourn.

In the "Before You Begin" section of the book, you filled out the "Where I've Come From" questionnaire. Today you will complete a similar questionnaire. The focus is on how you see yourself in relationship to God. You will revisit this questionnaire at the end of our thirty days together, by which time many changes will have occurred in the way you view yourself and God.

Now take a moment to reflect and do some truthful evaluation. Please resist the temptation to circle the answer that you wish were true. Be genuinely honest. No one will see this except you and a God who loves you.

On the following questions, circle the number that best applies.

1. I am comfortable with myself and my personality.

1	2	3	4	5	6	7	8	9	10
Never									Always

2. I am optimistic that I can change.

1	2	3	4	5	6	7	8	9	10
Never									Always

3. I have a tendency to put myself down or to call myself names.

1	2	3	4	5	6	7	8	9	10
Never									Always

4. I try to make others happy and to meet their expectations of me.

1	2	3	4	5	6	7	8	9	10
Never									Always

5. I derail my own goals.

1	2	3	4	5	6	7	8	9	10
Never									Always

6. I am self-conscious.

1	2	3	4	5	6	7	8	9	10
Never									Always

7. I feel I deserve to be put down by others.

1	2	3	4	5	6	7	8	9	10
Never									Always

8. My heart feels empty.

1	2	3	4	5	6	7	8	9	10
Never									Always

9. God is pleased with me.

1	2	3	4	5	6	7	8	9	10
Never									Always

10. I am angry at God.

1	2	3	4	5	6	7	8	9	10
Never									Always

11. I feel that God is angry with me.

1	2	3	4	5	6	7	8	9	10
Never									Always

12. God cares about how I feel.

1	2	3	4	5	6	7	8	9	10
Never									Always

13. I feel that God is reliable and trustworthy in my life.

1	2	3	4	5	6	7	8	9	10
Never									Always

14. I fear releasing my life completely to God.

1	2	3	4	5	6	7	8	9	10
Never									Always

15. God seems so distant.

1	2	3	4	5	6	7	8	9	10
Never									Always

16. I think God cares about my body and food issues.

1	2	3	4	5	6	7	8	9	10
Never									Always

17. I know God is there when I pray.

1	2	3	4	5	6	7	8	9	10
Never									Always

18. I think God forgives me.

1	2	3	4	5	6	7	8	9	10
Never									Always

19. I feel that I can confide in God.

1	2	3	4	5	6	7	8	9	10
Never									Always

20. I am aware of how God sees me, and I live my life accordingly.

1	2	3	4	5	6	7	8	9	10
Never									Always

21. I feel accepted and loved unconditionally by God.

1	2	3	4	5	6	7	8	9	10
Never									Always

22. I enjoy experiencing God's presence when I pray.

1	2	3	4	5	6	7	8	9	10
Never									Always

At the end of our thirty days together you will enjoy seeing how God has worked within you and how much you have changed. It is our prayer that by that time God will have revealed Himself to you in power and love and that you will find yourself more convinced that He is trustworthy. We pray that you will be amazed by His love and presence and more appreciative of the masterpiece that He crafted when He made you. Expect great things of Him. He will meet and surpass those expectations.

Amy, who reached her natural, God-given size says, "The initial Thin Within experience is incredibly freeing, and with the freedom comes a responsibility to be honest with God. When you are honest He meets you and true growth happens. Being a part of the program drove me into a deeper more satisfying relationship with God."

Let's risk a grander vision. Let's dare to have a look at the one who will lead us down this path to freedom. Who is God? What is He like? In whom do we place our faith? In whom are we asked to trust? Everything depends on our understanding of who He is, as we respond with our love, allegiance, and obedience.

God is love (1 John 4:8).

The most foundational of all the attributes of God is love. This attribute is so fundamental to His character that God uses it to describe Himself. His is an active love that has motivated all that He has done since the beginning of time. When He paints the evening sunset, it is because He loves you. When a child embraces you, it is because He loves you. When the birds sing, the sun rises, the flowers waft a heavenly scent, it is all because He loves you.

He was inspired to initiate relationships with human beings from the beginning of creation because it is in His character to love. He woos you and draws you, placing in you a desire to draw near to Him. That desire is kindled by His love for you. His word reminds us that we love Him only because He first loved us.

Our God is also amazingly creative. He is the one who formed the heavens, speaking the stars, the earth, the waters into existence. He shaped the varieties of living things that grace our planet and that are amazing to behold. Consider the duck-billed platypus. What fun the Lord must have had creating him! Or the porcupine, with his body covered with hollow, sharp hair called quills. A woodpecker has a skull especially made just for pounding the sides of trees and a tail with feathers designed to prop him up as he does his tap-tapping work. Consider the power God chose to place in the blue whale, or the fragrance of the most delicate orchid, the vines that cling to the great standing oak trees and the sweet juice that comes from wild berries. And He formed each of us so intricately to be a unique representation of His creativity.

Is he not . . . your Creator, who made you and formed you? (Deuteronomy 32:6b)

When we begin to see that God has created each one of us uniquely and very specifically, we begin to develop an appreciation for our own bodies. His divine imagination thought of you in eternity past and He created you especially for this space and this time. All of creation, including you, speaks of His wondrous glory.

The LORD is good and does what is right; he shows the proper path to those who go astray (Psalm 25:8, NLT).

God heard the prayer of the barren woman, who, in her culture would have been spurned for remaining childless. He gave Hannah the child for which she longed and prayed.

Simeon, an old prophet, prayed earnestly to see the Redeemer of Israel ushered into the world before his eyes closed in death. In answer to Simeon's prayer, one day as he served at the temple, God caused a young man and woman to present their firstborn son to Him for dedication. The child was called Jesus.

A hemorrhaging woman fell in the dust, longing only to touch Jesus' robe so that she could be healed. His power healed her instantly.

God selected a shepherd to be a king, a man with a lust problem to teach marital fidelity, a group of rough 'n' tumble guys to become great ministers of His gospel, and a Jewish Christian-killer to speak to Gentiles of new life in Jesus.

But you, O Lord, are a compassionate and gracious God, slow to anger, abounding in love and faithfulness (Psalm 86:15).

Grace, abundant and so free, flows from the throne of God. It envelops our thirsty souls and brings wonder and amazement to our lives. Our God is gracious indeed.

God's grace can be seen in the provision of the cloud by day and the pillar of fire by night, which He used to lead his people; in Jonah's deliverance from the whale after he had learned a difficult lesson about obedience; in the constant forgiveness of His people caught in a sin-repent-sin-repent cycle; in providing the sacrificial ram in the thicket for Isaac; in the selection of a young Jewish woman as the mother of the Messiah.

And, of course, as the ultimate sacrifice for our sins—yours and mine— we see Jesus, the perfect Lamb of God slain for us so we can have eternal life. Grace is abundant and free, flowing from the throne of our God. The God who offers this grace is the God who wants to be *your* constant companion on your journey to healing and wholeness. He offers you peace about your body and your relationship to food.

Rather than feeling condemned by others, yourself, and possibly even by God, our prayer is that you will lean on God's wonderful grace, which is available to you each moment of the day. One practical way you can enjoy the blessing of God's grace in an ongoing way and apply it freely to your Thin Within journey is through observation and correction.

The apostle Paul tells us, *We are hard pressed on every side, but not crushed; perplexed, but not in despair; persecuted, but not abandoned; struck down, but not destroyed* (2 Corinthians 4:8). God's grace allows us to rise each and every time we stumble on this path to freedom. We refrain from self-condemnation, and in the strength God provides, we adjust our actions. Through self-correction we continue to mature, growing ever closer to the heart of God and more in line with His desire for us. By His grace we wholeheartedly pursue holiness and by His grace He multiplies the effort one hundredfold.

As we begin to see God as creative, gracious, loving, and good, we develop a greater willingness to allow Him to direct our decisions and choices. It is in this place that we begin to appreciate the body He has created for us. Are you ready to listen to what God and your body have to say about your issues with eating and food?

Discovering My Own Hunger Level—The Bodometer Process

Since your body is one of God's masterpieces, it can be trusted. As you begin to believe that, you will also learn that your body can help guide you on your Thin Within journey as well. One way it will do that is by signaling you when it is hungry. Since Key #1 is to eat only when you are hungry, it is important to begin by defining just what we mean by "hungry."

Key #8 suggests that you stop at a point of comfort before you are full, so we will need a working definition of "full" as well. To do this, we are going to utilize a tool which we call the "bodometer process," that you can use at any time to check with your body about how hungry you actually are.

The Bodometer Process

To begin this process, sit in a comfortable chair with nothing on your lap. Invite God into the process. He will help make the answers clear to you.

Now focus your attention on your teeth. Sometimes people talk about "teeth hunger," which they describe as a need to chew. What do you experience in this area? Then focus your attention on your mouth. Are there any sensations in that area that you would call hunger? Any messages that say it is time to eat?

Now focus your attention on your throat. Are there any sensations there that you would call hunger? Time to eat? Comfortable? Stuffed? Any sensations of thirst in this area? Sometimes hunger is confused with a desire for liquids.

Now place your attention on your stomach, the area just below your rib cage. What sensations do you experience in this area? With what do you associate these sensations?

Next, move your attention to your lower abdomen. What sensations do you experience there? Do you have any hunger sensations in this part of your body? Often people think the stomach is located in both the upper and lower abdominal area when in fact it is just below your breastbone.

Finally, place your hands on the entire area of your stomach and abdomen. On a scale of 0 to 10—0 being empty, 5 being comfortable, and 10 being stuffed, at what level of hunger is your body right now? Write down that number. _____.

The sensations you may experience in your teeth, mouth, and throat are valid sensations, but that is not where you will experience true stomach hunger. You will want to refer to the area below your rib cage for an accurate indication of physiological hunger.

You will use the bodometer process frequently throughout our journey. This simple exercise is a way for you to tune out distractions and tune into your body.

We know that the one who created our bodies is wise. Therefore we can assume that our bodies are reliable and trustworthy. The hunger scale tool, which follows, then, will help you develop sensitivity to and trust of your body's signals.

The Hunger Scale Tool

One of the primary tools that we use in Thin Within is the Hunger Scale. We illustrate the various levels of hunger that you will experience this way:

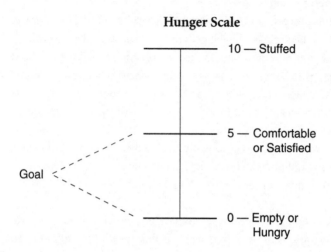

Hunger Scale

10 — Stuffed

5 — Comfortable or Satisfied

Goal

0 — Empty or Hungry

Remember that 0 is empty, 5 is comfortable, and 10 is stuffed. You know what we mean by stuffed—Thanksgiving-aching-belly-have-to-lie-down-on-the-sofa–can't-eat-another-bite stuffed.

At Thin Within when we say that we eat only when we're hungry and stop when we're comfortable, we mean 0 to 5 eating. There's no such thing as "I'm just a little bit hungry." You're either at a 0 or you're not. If you're not, you may be at a 1 or higher. We encourage you to eat only when you are clearly at 0. It's really that simple.

We can remove the anxiety from our eating when we reduce it down to this clear goal. Be encouraged that one of the things we're going to do during the next twenty-nine days is to help you bring your hunger numbers into clear focus. It may take some time to accomplish this but it will happen. As you trust the body that God has given you, and listen to the signals that it sends you, your hunger numbers will become much clearer.

You may be surprised at times to find that you're thirsty rather than hungry. What your body really wants is some cool, refreshing water. We highly recommend God's provision of water above any man-made beverage. Enjoy it in abundance. Always remember that the first key to conscious eating is eat only when your body is physically hungry—at a 0. If you consistently stop at 5, you will find the extra pounds seem to slide off of your body. If you start to eat when you are at a 3 on the hunger scale and stop at a 7, you will remain overweight. If you start to eat when you are at a 5 and continue until you are at 10, you will gain weight.

Hunger Scale

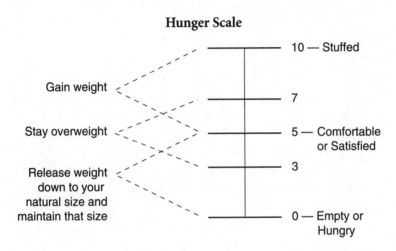

A surprising, yet little known fact is that your stomach when empty is about the size of your fist, which means that approximately a fist-sized amount of food is all that is required to take you from that 0 to a comfortable 5. That can be a great revelation to those who are accustomed to five-fisted eating; however, it is a reality, and when reckoned with can be quite freeing.

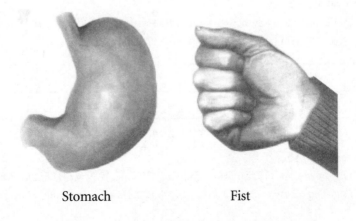

Stomach   Fist

To honor God, who walks with us, and who leads and directs us, we need to honor the unique and amazing body He has made especially for each of us. His word reminds us that we are fearfully and wonderfully made. And, as the saying goes, "God doesn't make junk." By eating from a 0 to 5, you will be on the path to the natural size He designed you to be.

Take Action

- Wait until you're hungry or at a 0 to eat.
- For the duration of this program, set aside your doubts and give your partnership with God a chance. You have nothing to lose but unwanted weight. In the space below, promise to give yourself the gift of freedom to become Thin Within. You might write something like, "I am not going to let my doubts keep me from this process. I will commit this approach to God one hundred percent as He leads me in ways of righteousness and truth." Feel free to express in your own words your desire to follow God.

_____

_____

_____

As we continue on our road to freedom, we can make the most of the tools that God has offered us. The hunger scale is merely that—a tool. Use it with prayerful discernment and you will find that it will be only a blessing to you as the Holy Spirit guides you and directs you.

Your Success Story

- Did you have any new insights while you were reading today? Please record them below.

_____

_____

_____

Verses to Ponder

Why do you say, O Jacob, and complain, O Israel, "My way is hidden from the LORD; my cause is disregarded by my God"? Do you not know? Have you not heard? The LORD *is the everlasting God, the Creator of the ends of the earth. He will not grow tired or weary, and His understanding no one can fathom. He gives strength to the weary and increases the power of the weak. Even youths grow tired and weary, and young men stumble and fall; but those who hope in the* LORD *will renew their strength. They will soar on wings like eagles; they will run and not grow weary, they will walk and not be faint* (Isaiah 40:27–31).

"*This is what the* LORD *says—your Redeemer, who formed you in the womb: I am the* LORD*, who has made all things, who alone stretched out the heavens, who spread out the earth by myself*" (Isaiah 44:24).

Prayer

Dear Lord, Please help me to know You better and to believe that You are good, compassionate, gracious, and a loving God. Help me to see You as You really are. Lord, I know at times that I haven't been waiting until I am truly hungry to eat. Help me to trust more in You and in the body You have given me. I thank You for the hope that I have found in You as I continue along this path toward wholeness. In Jesus' name I pray, Amen.

Medical Moment

From a physical viewpoint, our bodies are amazing. They are comprised of a dozen or so independent but interconnected organ systems working together under the control of a central computer, the brain, that receives a never-ending stream of information from inside and outside the body. It processes and utilizes this data to ensure the health of the body. And what wonderful bodies we have—with ears to hear music of the ages, eyes to behold the genius of a Rembrandt or a Michelangelo, and the gift of language, which allows us to enjoy the relationships so necessary for our lives.

—ARTHUR HALLIDAY, M.D.

Success Tools

+ Use the Thin Within Observations and Corrections Chart today.
+ To determine your hunger level, you may want to refer to the bodometer process.

✦ Use the Thin Within Keys to Conscious Eating when you choose to eat or drink today.

Thin Within Observations and Corrections Chart—Day 2

Observations	Day 2
1. I ate when my body was hungry.	
2. I ate in a calm environment by reducing distractions.	
3. I ate when I was sitting.	
4. I ate when my body and mind were relaxed.	
5. I ate and drank the things my body enjoyed.	
6. I paid attention to my food while eating.	
7. I ate slowly, savoring each bite.	
8. I stopped before my body was full.	

Thin Within Wisdom

God loves and accepts you just the way you are. You are *precious* to Him!

Going for Godly Goals

So we make it our goal to please him.
—2 Corinthians 5:9a

Yesterday we had a chance to get better acquainted with God, the one with whom we travel. We focused on the fact that God's nature is to love, that He is good, gracious, and has designed each body to be a unique representation of His amazing handiwork. For that reason no two people look exactly alike and no two paths to freedom will be identical. As we partner with God on this special road, our knowledge of Him will deepen and we will see that He is worthy of all of our trust. He is worthy to be followed, and He is most worthy to be adored.

As you listen and draw closer, you will hear God speak specifically to you about His plans for you—plans for a hope and a good future. And as you continue your journey, you will want your own vision, plans, and goals to line up with His. Our sincere desire is for you to experience the freedom for which you were created and to catch the vision that God has for your life. Today we will focus on the purpose of life and the blessing of adopting godly goals.

. . . everyone who is called by my name, whom I created for my glory, whom I formed and made (Isaiah 43:7).

God created us for His glory. He wants our lives to reflect His joy, love, grace, and compassion so that people will recognize Him in our countenance. The Bible calls this "glorifying God." You might say that we become advertisements for how wonderful God is when our lives display His majesty and wonder to the world.

Consider this example. What is a flashlight designed to do? Shine, of course, and when it is doing that for which it was designed, it does it well and effortlessly.

Now imagine the flashlight has feelings, thoughts, and emotions. It decides it doesn't want to do that for which it was created; it decides that it would rather be a hammer. But after pounding a few nails next to a real hammer how will the flashlight feel? Inadequate, ineffective, and beat-up, and eventually it will even fail to shine.

Many of us go through life not quite understanding what we were designed to do. We, too, may feel inadequate, ineffective, and beat-up. The good news is that this isn't God's plan for you! You can start today doing that for which you were created. You can choose to shine. And as you shine you will experience joy, freedom, rest, and peace. When you choose to glorify God, to make Him known, you are doing that for which you were created—"shining."

In the same way, let your light shine before men, that they may see your good deeds and praise your Father in heaven (Matthew 5:16).

Maureen, a Thin Within participant, rejoices in the way her God-given talents have been used since she began to see herself in light of His purposes. "The Lord began to reveal to me and others the gifts He had placed in me. Church leaders recognized my talents for dramatic skits. Needs arose for direction and writing and as I met those needs, I began to blossom. I don't think anyone really knew it, but these pursuits had been a dream of mine since I was a child. I was overjoyed to be able to express them in these small ways." God is reflected in Maureen's life as never before—in her body, in her countenance, and in her God-given gifts. When we shine for Him, we reflect God's love. Our light—or more accurately, God's light in us—attracts others.

In order to encourage you to shine in the way God intended, we invite you today to evaluate prayerfully the desires, gifts, talents, and experiences that God has brought together in your life. As you do this, we will ask you to create a vision statement. You will also be guided through a goal-setting activity. As you consider a godly vision and goals for your life, remain mindful that giving glory to God is the foundational purpose for your life.

For God knew his people in advance, and he chose them to become like his Son (Romans 8:29, NLT).

According to Psalm 139, God knew you and formed you in your mother's womb. When he designed you, He chose you to be like His Son. Jesus' life was lived with purpose and meaning. Jesus' character reflected all of the attributes of God.

For in Christ all the fullness of the Deity lives in bodily form (Colossians 2:9).

If we allow God to form and shape our character, we will become more like Jesus and we will live with rich purpose and meaning. Not only that, but if we allow Him to help us establish a godly vision and goals, it is through His power that we will attain them. He has a plan for us, and if we make His plan our plan, we will experience true success and boundless joy.

According to Charles Stanley, pastor and author, there are many benefits to setting godly goals:

1. Goals help you focus your efforts.
2. Goals help you set your schedule.
3. Goals help you balance your life.

Further, there are many godly characteristics and qualities that emerge in the person who has goals. This person . . .

1. has a direction in life.
2. has excitement about life.
3. has remarkable energy.
4. is often very creative.
5. pursues excellence.
6. has a great sense of appreciation for others who have goals.
7. tends to be physically healthier.
8. tends to be emotionally healthier.[1]

Sounds like a terrific deal, doesn't it? Take a moment to pray and invite God to help you capture His vision for your life. We will use the remainder of our time today in an activity that will help you see how God has gifted you and what vision and goals would exalt Him in your life. How has He uniquely made you to shine in your special way? Let's take a moment to pray together.

Lord, I really want to live according to Your purpose and plan for my life, but I am a bit fearful. Please help me to sense Your comfort and Your love as I put my trust in You. You have made me to shine in a special way. Help me to know what that is, Lord. Let me reflect your glory, in my body, my soul, and my spirit. In Jesus' name, I pray. Amen.

Vision Statement Exercise

Where there is no vision, the people perish (Proverbs 29:18, KING JAMES VERSION).

Consider prayerfully for a moment the talents, gifts, and desires you have. Also consider the things that you like to do. Consider, too, the fact that

God wants to use you to reach others. He wants to display His glory in you and through you. He wants you to become more like His son. Take a moment to pray. Ask God to help you see His vision for the unique qualities that make you who you are.

What would the tapestry of your life look like if you were to weave together all of the strands of talent, skill, gifts, and desires that God has placed in you? A vision statement may look something like this: *God has created me to bring His word alive so that people can experience His eternal truth in their everyday lives.*

An additional example might be: *God has created me to be a godly example of the love of Christ to widows and to the elderly.*

A vision is, by definition, somewhat broad. Now it's your turn.

_____

_____

_____

_____

Where Am I Going?—Realistic Goals Exercise

For each of the three goals you establish in this exercise, please follow Dr. Stanley's suggestions and for each one answer the following questions:

1. Why is this important to You, Lord?
2. Does this fit into Your plan for my life?
3. Is this goal totally in line with Your Word?
4. How might the accomplishment of this goal bring Your blessing to others?[2]

Kathy, who released twenty pounds during the program, reports, "As I began to pray and seek God regarding His vision and goals for my life, I was able to see that He had placed within me a longing to reach women with the word of truth. As I accepted the gifts, passions, desires, and talents God had given me as part of His plan to fulfill this life vision, I felt confidence to begin an Internet ministry that has been used of God to touch and encourage others."

In Romans 1:13 and 15:24, the apostle Paul tells the Roman Christians that he had planned to visit them on his way to a missionary trip in Spain.

One of his goals was to reach as many for Christ as He possibly could. He also planned to visit Corinth on his way to Macedonia. About this journey, Paul said something very intriguing to the Corinthian believers:

When I planned this, did I do it lightly? Or do I make my plans in a worldly manner so that in the same breath I say, "Yes, yes" and "No, no"? (2 Corinthians 1:17)

Paul clearly made a distinction between godly goal setting and worldly goal setting. We want to draw the same distinction and encourage you to invite God into this process. Remember that His primary purpose is for you to be more like Jesus and for you to glorify Him in body, soul, and spirit. Prayerfully consider each of the above questions as you make your goals consistent with the vision statement that you developed. While the vision is to be broad, goals can and should be more specific. The goals you set today are to be short-term goals, specifically for this period of time that you spend in *Thin Within*.

When you chose this book, you probably had a desire to be a different size than you are now. Even though you will be dealing with your weight, *Thin Within* is about much more than that. You will see that God's love and acceptance of you has nothing to do with your size. However, since we know that one of the ways we can bring God glory (make Him known to others) is by being our healthiest, it is reasonable to focus on making a concrete goal in this area. Ask God what size He designed you to be and state this as a godly goal. Keep in mind the fact that God's goals can be accomplished in the strength that He provides.

Goal #1: I believe that the Lord desires for me to release some excess weight. Therefore, after praying about it and inviting Him to indicate His will to me, my goal for Day Thirty is to be _____.

If anorexia or bulimia are areas where you are challenged, then use the following to establish an appropriate goal: *I believe that the Lord desires for me to be more attuned to His voice and to my God-given body.* After praying and seeking His direction, my goal for Day Thirty is to be _____.

Charles Stanley also encourages us to follow these principles when goal setting:

1. State precisely what you intend to accomplish (Mark 10:51).
2. Keep your goals private.
3. Set goals you can't reach on your own strength and ability.

4. Make a commitment to your goals
5. Take one step at a time.
6. Set a goal to successfully manage your success.
7. Take the plunge. "I'm going to take the risk. I'm going to jump in and see what happens."³

Make a second goal related to another area of your life that will support your dream of radiating health inside and out. Set a goal about which you can be enthusiastic, one that is not only honoring to God but also enjoyable.

Goal #2: I believe that the Lord desires for me to radiate health. Therefore, after praying to better understand His will for me, my goal for Day Thirty is _____. (Example: to exercise my body 15–30 minutes each day)

Now we ask you to take a bit more of a risk. Since our ultimate goal is to become more like Jesus, to see Him be glorified in and through us, how can you make God more widely known to those with whom you come in contact?

So often our dreams are too small while God's dreams for us are God-sized. When the apostle Paul became a Christian, his dream was to reach the Jews with the message of salvation. It was a great goal that seemed to be God-honoring, but it was too small. The Good News was spread across the entire world because God's goal for Paul was to reach the Gentiles. When Paul's goals were aligned with God's goals, the results were extraordinary and they changed history for all eternity.

Consider carefully what might be a God-sized goal for you. Really stretch yourself, remembering that you will have twenty-eight days to accomplish it. As an idea, consider your environment. Many who have struggled with chaotic eating seem to have disorder in other areas of their lives as well. Why not step out on a limb and, with God's help, conquer some of the "land," something specific in your life? If your home isn't of concern to you, what about your job or your church or your neighborhood? Is there some way in which you could make inroads in any of these areas, trusting God in a new fresh way? For example, you might step out in faith and join the choir or visit an elderly person each week. You might make a point to keep your desktop clear of clutter or to shelve all the books sitting in boxes from the job change you made two years ago. You decide.

**Goal #3 I believe that the Lord desires for me to_____
by Day Thirty in the strength that He provides.**

*The steps of the godly are directed by the LORD. He delights in every detail
of their lives* (Psalm 37:23, NLT).

Now, restate your three goals below so that you can more easily refer to
them.

**Goal #1 By God's grace and the strength I will to be in a dress or belt
size _____ by Day Thirty.**

**Goal #2 By God's grace and the strength I will _____
_____ by Day Thirty.**

**Goal #3 By God's grace and the strength I will _____
_____ by Day Thirty.**

God delights in every detail of your life. In fact, we believe that the
process you are going through right now brings honor and glory to Him. It
is a wonderful thing to be invited by the Lord to participate in the plans He
has for you, for His people, and for His world. As we purpose together in
our hearts to live according to a godly vision and goals, we discover that
there is much more to life than we previously imagined.

Take Action

- ✦ Wait until you are hungry, at a 0 to eat.
- ✦ Throughout the day, reread your goals to get more focused on what
  God wants you to accomplish. As you do this, pray that God will help
  you to achieve them.

Your Success Story

Did you have any new insights while you were reading today? Please
record them below.

_____

_____

_____

Verses to Ponder

*I consider that our present sufferings are not worth comparing with the
glory that will be revealed in us* (Romans 8:18).

So whether you eat or drink or whatever you do, do it all for the glory of God
(1 Corinthians 10:31).

And we, who with unveiled faces all reflect the Lord's glory, are being trans-
formed into his likeness with ever-increasing glory, which comes from the Lord,
who is the Spirit (2 Corinthians 3:18).

Prayer

Dear Lord, thank You that I can set godly goals and have Your strength to
draw on in order to accomplish them. I pray that You will help me perse-
vere. I want to bring You honor and to cause others to hunger and thirst
for You as they see Your glory reflected in me. In the name of Jesus, Amen.

Medical Moment

The health of Americans is suffering greatly because of an epidemic
that continues to escalate. The good news is that it is one hundred percent preventable and one hundred percent curable. What is it? This
epidemic is overeating. The solution is eating the way a naturally thin
person eats, a person who is not obsessed with dieting and exercise.
We invite you to enter into this exciting approach as it works for everyone. I can personally attest to this, having seen many of my patients
over the past eighteen years experience dramatic health improvements
after applying this "cure."

—ARTHUR HALLIDAY, M.D.

Success Tools

+ Wait until you are at a 0 before eating.
+ If you are eating beyond your "comfort" level, then consider eating
  one-half or one-third of your usual portion. Give yourself twenty
  minutes to digest that amount of food and see if you aren't at that
  comfortable 5 on your hunger scale.
+ Use the Thin Within Observations and Corrections Chart today.
+ You may refer to the bodometer process in Day Two as a way of determining your hunger level before you eat.
+ Use the Thin Within Keys to Conscious Eating when you choose to eat
  or drink today.

Thin Within Observations and Corrections Chart—Day 3

Observations	Day 3
1. I ate when my body was hungry.	
2. I ate in a calm environment by reducing distractions.	
3. I ate when I was sitting.	
4. I ate when my body and mind were relaxed.	
5. I ate and drank the things my body enjoyed.	
6. I paid attention to my food while eating.	
7. I ate slowly, savoring each bite.	
8. I stopped before my body was full.	

Thin Within Wisdom

Try for nothing and hit it every time. Set godly goals and watch what God will do!

NOTES

1. Charles Stanley, *Success God's Way: Achieving True Contentment And Purpose* (Nashville, Tennessee: Thomas Nelson, Inc., 2000), 33–34.
2. ibid, 46.
3. ibid, 53–58.

A Path of My Choosing

You have made known to me the path of life;
you will fill me with joy in your presence,
with eternal pleasures at your right hand.
—Psalm 16:11

God showers His love upon us—a love that is better than life. It is our privilege to glorify and praise Him all the days we walk upon the earth. In this we are filled with joy and find eternal pleasure in the presence of Almighty God. No food can even begin to compare with the satisfaction that comes from basking in His presence. No drink can quench the thirst of the soul crying out for the Lord.

As the deer pants for streams of water, so my soul pants for you, O God. My soul thirsts for God, for the living God. When can I go and meet with God? (Psalm 42:1–2)

In spite of our own thirsting souls, we typically don't cling to the Lord moment by moment of every day. Although our wandering disrupts our fellowship with Him, the breech in intimacy need not last long. Thankfully God has provided for our waywardness on our Thin Within journey with the tool we call "observation and correction." Many of our workshop participants have found this simple principle to be life changing. Jenny writes, "Grace fills my life now that I have learned that I don't need to punish myself for my mistakes. I can acknowledge my errors and then accept the forgiveness that God offers, allowing His grace to wash over me as I correct my behavior. It has revolutionized my approach to life and obedience."

Here is how this principle works. At any given point in time, you can choose to note any behaviors, beliefs, and attitudes that haven't worked for you. For instance, upon reading the keys to conscious eating in Day One, John decided that he would wait until he was definitely hungry before eating. On Day Two, however, he got up early and ate breakfast because he was hungry, went to work and before he knew it had eaten several donuts from the coffee lounge. He then realized that he hadn't given a single thought to hunger before devouring the donuts.

John can choose to take note of his behavior: "Hmm. I saw the donuts on the counter and they looked so good, that without checking with the Lord or even thinking about hunger, I inhaled them." That is observation. To get the most out of the tool of observation and correction, John will withhold any self-condemnation. Let's illustrate it as he watches himself on a TV screen. Please refer to figure 4-1.

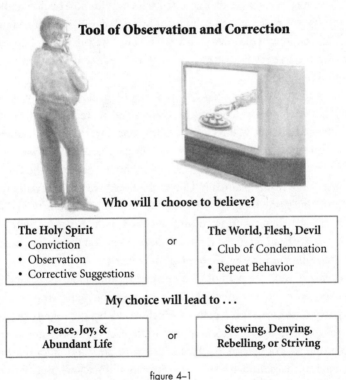

Tool of Observation and Correction

Who will I choose to believe?

The Holy Spirit		The World, Flesh, Devil
• Conviction	or	• Club of Condemnation
• Observation		• Repeat Behavior
• Corrective Suggestions		

My choice will lead to ...

Peace, Joy, & Abundant Life	or	Stewing, Denying, Rebelling, or Striving

figure 4–1

If he applies the tool of observation and correction the way it is intended, John looks upon this imaginary TV screen objectively. He can then choose one of two differing perspectives. He can choose to respond to the voice of the Holy Spirit. Or he can listen to the accusing tones of the world, his own flesh, or the Enemy, Satan.

Let's assume that John chooses to listen to the Holy Spirit. This enables him to observe his behavior for the purpose of bringing about conviction and godly correction. In this place there is no self-condemnation (Romans 8:1). There is grace, abundant and *free*. John observes in the power of the Holy Spirit and is convicted. He makes alterations to correct the behavior (donut eating) that didn't coincide with his goals of using the keys to conscious eating (eating only when hungry). Rather than think poorly of himself for what he did an hour ago, he identifies what he can do to avoid the same behavior again. Then he simply changes his behavior, making these corrections in the present moment.

It is simple—so simple that we often miss it. With observation and correction there is peace, joy, and abundant living. We walk in faith and in the grace of God, not in our own ability to pull ourselves up by our bootstraps or to whip ourselves into shape. We walk in dependence on God in each present moment.

This is illustrated in figure 4-2. If you choose to allow the Holy Spirit to bring conviction and apply the observation and correction tool, you will find life is stabilized by the cross of Christ and covered by the canopy of grace. You will look to God for provision for your needs. What would otherwise be a life of extremes is now stabilized by the power of the Cross. It becomes a life firmly planted in Christ, the Rock. We call this walking the "path of God's provision." As we continue on this path, we may find ourselves going two steps forward and one step back. However, without a doubt, we are heading in the right direction. We are on the path to holiness and the abundant life we have been given in Christ.

When you walk the path of God's provision, your focus is on God. You will experience the way in which He inspires, enables, and empowers you every step of the way. It is a path on which we are being progressively conformed to the image of Christ. We rest in the fact that God knows we are flawed, and we praise Him that He has provided the solution for our problem. He loves us so much and wants absolute intimacy with us. *While we were still sinners, Christ died for us* (Romans 5:8).

On this path God's canopy of grace shelters us during the storms of life and shades us during those days when we experience fiery trials. If we attempt to move out from under God's protective covering, we quickly discover that life consists of frustration and striving and goes nowhere. As we choose to surrender to God and His wonderful care for us, we experience His peace and His sufficiency. We learn that He truly is satisfying, more than the richest of foods. The perfecting power of the Holy Spirit works from the inside out—from within. He gives us a new mind and a new heart, not a new formula.

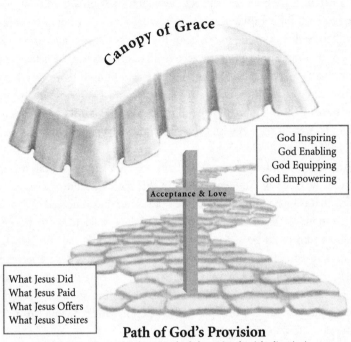

Canopy of Grace

God Inspiring
God Enabling
God Equipping
God Empowering

Acceptance & Love

What Jesus Did
What Jesus Paid
What Jesus Offers
What Jesus Desires

Path of God's Provision
(Two steps forward and one step back, but going the right direction)

figure 4–2

On the path of God's provision under the canopy of His grace, at any moment we can run into the loving arms of Abba, Father. If we find ourselves diving face first into a bag of Oreos, we can stop, observe, and call out to the Lord who answers us in our distress. Applying His grace, we can correct and move on, experiencing and receiving the fullness of God's forgiveness. The tool of observation and correction enables us to acknowledge that we have made mistakes. We identify those mistakes and agree with God that they are sin. We can then turn back to Him in repentance and move forward, assured that our spirit has been washed "white as snow" (Isaiah 1:18).

Without this simple tool of observation and correction, John would see himself from another perspective. In looking back at the first illustration with the TV screen, he would listen to the world, the flesh (his natural man, who still has an influence even though he is a believer), or even Satan. These voices will attempt to influence his behavior and decisions.

Rather than observe and correct, he might dwell on what he saw, condemn himself for it, rant and rave about it, deny it or eat even more because of it. Rather than heeding the voice of the Spirit, which would bring godly correction, John would allow the accuser to have his way. If he listens to the world, his flesh, or the enemy, he may convince himself that everything is going wrong in his life. As he strives harder and harder, his resentment builds. He might even slip into all out rebellion. That is not a place he wants to find himself. It certainly isn't the abundant holy life we have been given in Christ.

John may beat himself up emotionally. At Thin Within we call this getting out the "club of condemnation." In this place of failure, John is convinced that if he had just "tried harder," he would have succeeded. He may end up thinking that he should just throw in the towel and accept defeat. If he allows himself to get stuck, he will feel that the only way out is to turn the keys to conscious eating into rigid rules, which they were never intended to become, and when that doesn't work he may swing to the other extreme of no self-control, or license. This pendulum-swinging lifestyle is reflected in what we call the "path of my performance." Living this way is falling into the trap of the legalist.

In this situation self is actually the focus rather than God. Even if the person is a believer, he or she will think that the solution to any failure is to "try harder." This struggler is always searching for the next book, the next program, the next church service, to find the "key" to success. What is missing, of course, is the grace of God and the power of the Holy Spirit enabling us to "observe and correct."

The truth is, grace isn't missing at all. It just hasn't been fully embraced. Those who find themselves in this predicament are like thirsty travelers who are unaware of a nearby fountain of life-giving water. The legalist swings from feeling good about her accomplishments on the one hand, to realizing that she can't keep up the pace on the other hand. Eventually she just gives up altogether, seeing herself as a "failure." Self-loathing sets in and she wallows in guilt, self-condemnation, self-pity, and sin. Before long, she goes out in search of another diet, another regimen, another set of rules. This is illustrated in figure 4-3.

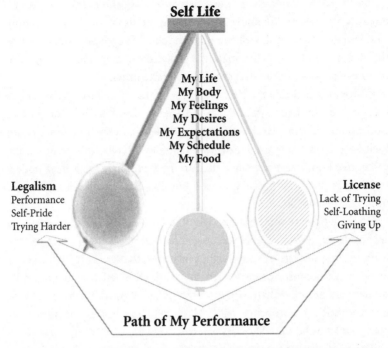

Self Life

My Life
My Body
My Feelings
My Desires
My Expectations
My Schedule
My Food

Legalism
Performance
Self-Pride
Trying Harder

License
Lack of Trying
Self-Loathing
Giving Up

Path of My Performance

figure 4–3

Thankfully there is an antidote to this pendulum pandemonium. There is hope! There is no reason to stay stuck. Our God is willing and He is able. If you find yourself on the path of your performance, you can jump ship into an ocean of grace, deeper than any sin, broader than any transgression. It is cool, refreshing, and free. It cost our Savior everything, but in His love He offers it freely to us.

How do you move from the path of your performance to the path of God's provision? How do we change this futile process into one of constant maturity in our Lord and Savior Jesus Christ? In matters of food and eating, the key is to move steadily forward with a sincere heart of willingness and faith, allowing yourselves to observe and correct your behavior. You may not like what you see, but ask yourself, "What really is the worst thing that can happen if I confess that I ate when I wasn't hungry and I didn't stop when I was satisfied?"

We only deceive ourselves by our lack of honesty and harm ourselves by our lack of progress. We know the truth. Our bodies know it and certainly God knows it. We may as well eliminate the club of condemnation and state the obvious. "I blew it." Then make the godly correction. "Thank you, Lord, that I can press on in the strength that You have provided."

Colleen learned this the hard way. "I was heavily involved in a weight-loss program for five years and lost 105 pounds. But I always thought that God would withdraw His love from me if I blew it. Every time I messed up I felt I was a big fat disappointment to Him." Eventually Colleen found the grace, freedom, and acceptance that are hers in Christ. She now understands that sin is not pleasing to God but that His love is not withdrawn from us when we do sin.

Once we observe our behavior, with the Lord's leading and strength we are able to apply godly correction. As I explained this principle to a participant, she responded, "It seems right but it isn't that easy." It isn't easy for many of us because we have lived for years with self-ridicule and self-condemnation rather than with the truth of God's Word. We have to break free from such lies, realizing that God doesn't condemn us. He does however, convict us because He loves us.

Therefore, there is now no condemnation for those who are in Christ Jesus (Romans 8:1).

Diane, a Thin Within participant points out: "Just as with my quiet time with God, I can get off track. But I always gently bring myself back. There's a lot of grace involved because we all stumble along the way. I still make mistakes, like eating something someone offers me even if I don't want it or if I'm not hungry. Now I'm learning to say, 'No thank you, I'm not hungry,' or to ask, 'Can I take it home?'

"I also use the 'observe' and 'correct' tool even in situations not related to food, such as dealing with parents and my students. I ask myself, 'What could I have done differently to produce a better outcome?'"

If you ask yourself this same question, you will be amazed at how quickly you can learn, grow, and mature on the path of God's provision. Put away your club of condemnation. Instead, experience God's grace in action with the principle of observation and correction.

Don, who applied this principle, shares, "Thin Within has helped me build my life in the present. It freed me to enjoy and praise God while in process, rather than waiting until I had achieved my goal." Don recognizes that we all fall short of the glory of God (Romans 3:23) and that none of us is perfect this side of heaven. Yet with the power of the Holy Spirit we can move onward and forward, one courageous step at a time.

As a father has compassion on his children, so the LORD has compassion on those who fear him; for he knows how we are formed, he remembers that we are dust (Psalm 103:13–14).

On the path of God's provision we see that His love reaches out beyond anything we can fathom. It is vast and deep. Psalm 36:5–6 says, *Your love, O LORD, reaches to the heavens, your faithfulness to the skies. Your righteousness is like the mighty mountains, your justice like the great deep.* On the path of my performance we constantly doubt we have "won" His love or approval.

Along the course of our journey we are beginning to see that our God is a God of power. He is able. He is good. And He can take our humble failings, as we offer them to Him, *causing even the worst of them to work for good, as we love Him and are called according to His purposes* (Romans 8:28).

Take Action

+ Commit to waiting until you are hungry before you eat. Your food will be much more enjoyable.

+ Consider the two paths cited above and take a moment to evaluate which path you are on. Ask yourself if your value comes from your accomplishments or from the one who created you. Is your desire to be, to do, or to have more? Is your focus on following your will or God's will? Record your thoughts.

_____

_____

_____

+ The chart that follows allows you to apply the tool of observation and correction. See if you can come up with a way to correct some observed behavior that doesn't bring about the desired results. The first one is done for you.

Enjoy the privilege today of applying God's grace in the present moment. You don't need to wallow in any measure of self-contempt. Observe what hasn't worked, agree with God, correct your behavior in the strength He gives you. Then move on down the path of God's provision as you experience the abundant life.

What You Have Observed	How You Will Correct
Example: 1. I have just made my way through half a bag of Oreos after my stressful day at work. I don't feel any better than when I started. Now I am feeling depressed and even more stressed.	*Example:* Next time I will put my feet up for a bit or take a hot bath. I could even try a 15-minute nap or a walk around the neighborhood.
2. I went to the buffet after church and ate too much and now I am stuffed. I always seem to do that when I go to the buffet.	
3. I just ate my way through two bags of microwave popcorn and I have no memory of it. The movie was great, but I always seem to bring out the food when I turn on a video.	
4. Whenever I go out to dinner with Barbara we eat a whole pizza together.	
5. I went to my mom's house and later realized I had snacked for the whole hour I was there.	

Your Success Story

Record below any new insights while you were reading today.

_____

_____

_____

Verses to Ponder

The LORD is my shepherd, I shall not be in want. He makes me lie down in green pastures, he leads me beside quiet waters, he restores my soul. He guides me in paths of righteousness for his name's sake (Psalm 23:1–3).

I run in the path of your commands, for you have set my heart free (Psalm 119:32).

The path of the righteous is like the first gleam of dawn, shining ever brighter till the full light of day (Proverbs 4:18).

Prayer

Thank You, Lord, that I don't have to beat myself up when I make mistakes. Help me to observe my behavior, and to correct it when it doesn't line up with the goals I have prayerfully set with You. Help me to recognize more clearly what hunger really feels like and to be aware of the hunger signals my body sends to me. When I am in doubt help me to pause, ask You, and trust the answer I receive. Give me patience to wait until I am truly hungry before I eat. Thank You for being with me on this exciting journey. In Jesus' name, Amen.

Medical Moment

All food is a gift and there are no forbidden foods unless:

1. There is a true food allergy.

2. There is a medical condition proscribing certain foods.

3. There is a potential drug/food interaction.

Certainly foods vary widely in their nutritious value, but most of our eating problems result from overeating. Chocolate-chip cookies or a donut, while less nutritious than salads, veggies, fish, lean meats, etc., are only bad for us if we overindulge.

What has been demonstrated through research projects is that when we accept that there are no forbidden foods, when we check in with our bodies to determine true hunger, and when we use the Thin Within Keys to Conscious Eating, we gradually shift to making wiser and healthier food choices. The payoff, especially if weight is released, is wonderful. We see improvement in a whole variety of medical conditions including hypertension, diabetes, cholesterol levels, better breathing and digestive function, as well as more energy, not to mention emotional, psychological, and spiritual well-being.

—ARTHUR HALLIDAY, M.D.

Success Tools

- ✦ Wait until you are at a 0 before eating.
- ✦ Use the Thin Within Observations and Corrections Chart.
- ✦ Use the bodometer process before you eat.
- ✦ Use the Thin Within Keys to Conscious Eating when you choose to eat or drink.

Thin Within Observations and Corrections Chart—Day 4

Observations	Day 4
1. I ate when my body was hungry.	
2. I ate in a calm environment by reducing distractions.	
3. I ate when I was sitting.	
4. I ate when my body and mind were relaxed.	
5. I ate and drank the things my body enjoyed.	
6. I paid attention to my food while eating.	
7. I ate slowly, savoring each bite.	
8. I stopped before my body was full.	

Thin Within Wisdom

Rejoice in the grace of our God.

Put away the club of condemnation.

❦

My Body, Fearfully and Wonderfully Made

Your hands shaped me and made me. . . .
You molded me like clay.
—Job 10:8–9

On Day Four, we saw that God's steadfast love and acceptance are totally unconditional. Our performance is not the key. His choice to love us is. We can, in fact, view each of our mistakes—each of our weaknesses—as an opportunity to witness God's hand at work.

But he said to me, "My grace is sufficient for you, for my power is made perfect in weakness." Therefore I will boast all the more gladly about my weaknesses, so that Christ's power may rest on me. That is why, for Christ's sake, I delight in weaknesses, in insults, in hardships, in persecutions, in difficulties. For when I am weak, then I am strong (2 Corinthians 12:9–10).

Aware of this, we step into the light of God's boundless, unconditional love. As we lift our heads we hear Him sing:

Listen, O daughter, consider and give ear: Forget your people and your father's house. The king is enthralled by your beauty; honor him, for he is your Lord (Psalm 45:10–11).

What an amazing and healing truth! As we take God at His word, we can rest in the fact that He treasures us. If we fail to do so, we live our lives "trying to measure up" assuming that God's approval depends on our performance. We never quite feel we have truly arrived, so we may even become angry with ourselves and even with God. This is no way to live, especially not for those who are on a quest for freedom. If this cycle continues, it drives us to endless striving that results in a lack of peace and a lack of progress.

On the other hand, the more we are able to accept His love, the more we will be able to assume the roles that He has designed for us. This may be difficult for us to believe, but as Maggie, another Thin Within participant, says, "God loves me no matter what and accepts me even when I sin. Sin breaks my fellowship with Him, but not my relationship."

We all come to God as we are, knowing that we all have dark closets that we would rather keep hidden. But out of His profound love, He waits for us to offer Him the keys to those closets, to admit that we can't manage life in our own strength. So we give ourselves to God, broken and humble, bleeding and torn, hopes dashed and hearts rent. This is a moment set in eternity past—the moment for which we were destined, when we humbly take His gift of complete forgiveness for all the times we refused to answer His call. We choose to surrender all, though it may not seem like much, and allow Him to shower us with all of the mercy, grace, forgiveness, and love that He longs to give us. He receives us to Himself with joy and gladness beyond our comprehension.

Yet to all who received him, to those who believed in his name, he gave the right to become children of God—children born not of natural descent, nor of human decision or a husband's will, but born of God (John 1:12).

Jesus taught that when we are born anew by the Spirit, we enter into God's family and are adopted as His precious children (John 3:3). From that moment on, His Holy Spirit, the very presence of God, comes to reside in our hearts. By His divine choice we are made heirs of God and co-heirs with Christ (Romans 8:17).

Therefore, if anyone is in Christ, he is a new creation; the old has gone, the new has come (2 Corinthians 5:17).

Through faith God Himself has come to be present within you. He has entrusted something very precious to you by pouring Himself into your life. All the love, joy, and delight He has in you are yours to experience as you rest in His embrace.

But we have this treasure [the presence of God] *in jars of clay to show that this all-surpassing power is from God and not from us* (2 Corinthians 4:7).

The jar of clay referred to in this passage is you. It is your body and your soul (mind, emotions, will, and feelings). We are vessels, containers of the life of God. But we are not the contents of the vessel. God is. We cannot produce His life, but we can reflect it. The beauty and value of the vessel is found in what it contains. We continue to be transformed more and more as we look to God rather than to ourselves.

But we all, looking on the glory of the Lord, with unveiled face, are transformed according to the same image from glory to glory (2 Corinthians 3:18, DARBY).

You are a work in progress. In fact, the Lord calls you His poetry. You are

His poetry in motion, His masterpiece (Ephesians 2:10). He has created you with a purpose. This is what Louise, who formerly struggled with anorexia and bulimia, accurately calls "grace—profound, transforming, life-producing grace."

During this next exercise we want to encourage you to look at yourself through the eyes of God. How does He view you? We hope that the last four days have laid a foundation of truth for you. Now we are ready to build on that foundation, but first we want to offer you a tool that, as you progress, will allow you to measure physical changes that occur on this journey.

Mirror, Mirror Exercise

Many who have struggled with food and body issues avoid looking at themselves in the mirror because of the shame they feel about their bodies. Others may realize that their reluctance to look in the mirror is due to some physical "difference" that God has allowed, something that seems to set them apart from other people. However, today keep in mind just how amazing your body is. No matter what your situation, your body has been created in intricate detail. Our prayer is that you might see yourself in a new light. You are a vessel, precious in God's sight, set apart to carry His presence.

The reason we ask you to look carefully at your body today is because by the end of this thirty-day period your body will change and you will want to have an accurate recollection of where you began.

One Thin Within participant named Marge says, "I went years not really looking at my body. I was molested repeatedly by my father when I was a child and was embarrassed by the fact that I was a woman. I went years trying to hide my femininity behind extra weight and when I finally did look in a mirror, I was shocked at what I saw. I was filled with even more shame and I resolved not to look anymore.

"When I was asked to do the Mirror, Mirror Exercise," Marge continued, "the thought of it turned my stomach. I agreed to do it, skeptical that anything good could result. I tried to discipline myself to look in the mirror and to praise God for my body. Boy, was that difficult! I was so surprised that only three weeks into the program, I not only began to accept what I saw, but I also began to be genuinely thankful for my body. Not only that, but there really were visible physical changes. I was so eager to tell my husband and my sister that I had, for the first time in my adult life, become reconciled to my own body. Talk about a miracle."

We hope that you make a discovery as wonderful as Marge's. Please try to withhold judgment and be a compassionate observer. Give praise to the Lord by honoring the body that He has given you. If this exercise becomes challenging for you at any moment, stop and pray, thanking and praising God for the many blessings He has given you. Then, when you are ready, resume the exercise. Are you ready? Praying for perseverance is certainly allowed.

Begin by standing in front of a mirror. We are aware of the fact that some people cannot stand because of physical limitations. My beloved friend Jeneka, who was born without legs, attended the workshop and openly expressed her heartfelt anger and disappointment with God regarding her disability. She said, "God and I have really wrestled it out over this one. However, over the years He has given me eyes to see beauty among ashes, and I can now praise Him for how my physical limitation has kept me dependent on Him."

We encourage you to allow the love of Christ to fall afresh on you as you come to the mirror. Please do whatever will allow you to enter into this exercise to the best of your ability. Observe your entire body and see yourself as God sees you. Take a moment to praise God that you are fearfully and wonderfully made. Imagine what it must have been like in the garden of Eden where they *were both naked, and they felt no shame* (Genesis 2:25). What freedom that must have been! That is, of course, what God intended.

Withholding all judgment, look at yourself from head to toe, front to back. If you notice yourself becoming critical, filled with shame, or evaluating yourself negatively, refute the thought with God's truth: "I am fearfully and wonderfully made."

Do this slowly, looking carefully at each part. First notice your toes and feet. What sensations do you feel in your feet? How have they served you over the years? Thank God for your feet, which have carried you through life.

Take a moment to look at the your legs below your knees. How do you feel about your calves? They work hard to move you from step to step, so take a moment to thank God for your calves.

Knees are marvelous works of machinery. Look at your knees and bend your legs, each in turn. What sensations do you have in your knees? How have they served you? Take a moment to give praise to God for the amazing work displayed in your knees.

Now notice your upper legs. Touch your legs. How do they feel? How have your upper legs served you? The muscles in this part of your body may be very strong. Thank God for your upper legs and the way they have served you so faithfully.

Continue observing your hips and buttocks. What sensations are you aware of in this area? How have your hips and buttocks served you? Give gratitude to God for your hips and buttocks.

Now become aware of your stomach and abdomen. Feel this part of your body. What do you notice? Thank God for the way your stomach has served you.

Turn your attention to your chest and rib cage. What sensations are you aware of? How do you feel about your chest and rib cage? Take a moment to express your appreciation for your chest and rib cage.

Relax your arms and let them hang at your sides and take a deep breath. Look at your arms and notice how you feel about them. Consider all the tasks that your arms and hands have enabled you to accomplish through your life. Think about the play, the work, the hugs, the serving of others. Thank God for your arms and hands.

Become aware of your shoulders and the area between your shoulder blades. What sensations do you have in this area? Is that part of your body tight or relaxed? If you feel tight, raise your arms and move them around to try to loosen up your shoulders. Move your head forward gently, down, side to side. Do you feel more relaxed? How have your shoulders and back served you during your life? Thank God for your shoulders and back.

Now focus your attention on your face. Touch your face, the area under your chin, your neck, and your hair. How has your face served you? Consider all of the expressions it is able to convey. Take a moment to praise God for your face.

Consider again that you are God's unique creation, fearfully and wonderfully made. You may not look quite the way you want to, but you are an amazing masterpiece nonetheless. Let's rest in the fact that He who has begun a great, marvelous work in you will carry it on to completion (Philippians 1:6).

Take Action

+ Use the space below to record your observations and thoughts that surfaced during the Mirror, Mirror Exercise.

_____

_____

_____

✦ Commit afresh to waiting until your body is at a 0 before eating.

Even now God is doing an amazing thing in the process you are undergoing. Thank you for allowing yourself to be led by God for these past four days. Consider what this says about you. It means that you have a heart hungering for the Lord. You desire His truth, His change, His will in your life. You are availing yourself to the will of your Maker. You are precious in His sight and He continues to form you and perfect you. You are His masterpiece. You are His poetry in motion. He has chosen you, and you belong to Him. Rejoice, fellow traveler. Our journey is just underway and there is much adventure ahead!

Your Success Story

Did you have any new insights while you were reading today? Please record them below.

_____

_____

_____

Verses to Ponder

For you created my inmost being; you knit me together in my mother's womb. I praise you because I am fearfully and wonderfully made; your works are wonderful, I know that full well. My frame was not hidden from you when I was made in the secret place. When I was woven together in the depths of the earth, your eyes saw my unformed body. All the days ordained for me were written in your book before one of them came to be (Psalm 139:13–16).

Yet, O LORD, you are our Father. We are the clay, you are the potter; we are all the work of your hand (Isaiah 64:8).

Prayer

Dear Lord, I know that I am fearfully and wonderfully made but sometimes I don't feel like it. You made me so that I could contain a wonder-

ful treasure—You. O, Lord, I pray that I might see myself as You see me. There are many things about my body that I hope to change, but even now I accept my privileged role as the temple of the Holy Spirit. Continue Your work in and through me, and I pray that the changes on the inside will become visible on the outside. Most importantly I pray that Your joy and love will flow through me to others. In Jesus' name, Amen.

Medical Moment

Each of the seventy-five to one hundred trillion cells that make up our bodies must be nourished twenty-four hours a day. Our intestinal tract, which is twenty to twenty-five feet long, is programmed to extract the necessary vitamins, minerals, carbohydrates, proteins, and fats from our diets for proper fueling, maintenance, and repair of all the body's tissues. Energy consumed in excess of the day's needs is stored as fat for use when food intake is limited, and what is not usable is excreted by the colon. The cardiovascular system delivers nourishment to every cell in the body and removes waste products, which are then excreted by the lungs and kidneys. To accomplish this the heart must pump about five quarts of blood, beating sixty to seventy times per minute—100,000 beats per day, about forty million times per year. Consider the musculoskeletal system—206 bones and hundreds of muscles, tendons, and ligaments, which allow for the most delicate movements of the fingers of the artist to the most Herculean feats of world-class athletes.

We are truly, "fearfully and wonderfully made."

—ARTHUR HALLIDAY, M.D.

Success Tools

+ Commit to waiting until you are hungry to eat.
+ Use the Thin Within Observations and Corrections Chart today.
+ Use the Thin Within Keys to Conscious Eating when you choose to eat or drink today.

Thin Within Observations and Corrections Chart—Day 5

Observations	Day 5
1. I ate when my body was hungry.	
2. I ate in a calm environment by reducing distractions.	
3. I ate when I was sitting.	
4. I ate when my body and mind were relaxed.	
5. I ate and drank the things my body enjoyed.	
6. I paid attention to my food while eating.	
7. I ate slowly, savoring each bite.	
8. I stopped before my body was full.	

Thin Within Wisdom

Praise God for your body. It is fearfully and wonderfully made. You are His masterpiece.

My Body, God's Temple

He will be the sure foundation for your times,
a rich store of salvation and wisdom and knowledge.
—Isaiah 33:6

So far this week we have been laying a foundation upon which we will continue to build over the next twenty-four days. As we see in Isaiah 33:6, the true foundation of our lives is Christ. We have been seeking Him so that our foundation is not an illusion of reality, but the solid rock of the Living Word.

Yesterday we saw our bodies as jars of clay, made priceless by the contents within. Some of us may truly appreciate the image of the clay pot when we consider the condition of our bodies. Perhaps we see ourselves as being very ordinary. Maybe we even think we are "cracked" pots. There is some truth in this imagery; however, we shouldn't let this perspective carry us to a place where we view our bodies with little or no regard.

God doesn't see us that way. He knows that a plain pot carrying a priceless treasure has great value. To be sure that we don't depart from a godly humility into a place of self-deprecation over this clay pot image, God has also spoken to us through the imagery of His temple in referring to our bodies.

Do you not know that your body is a temple of the Holy Spirit, who is in you, whom you have received from God? (1 Corinthians 6:19a)

To capture a sense of God's view of each of us, let's consider the places where God has chosen to dwell on earth. Some thirty-five-hundred years ago, God gave specifications for Moses to build a tabernacle in the wilderness. He provided highly detailed instructions and He gifted craftsmen to accomplish the work with mastery and grandeur. This tabernacle was to travel with the people as they wandered through the desert. God has always wanted to dwell among His people, and He always did it in style. The tabernacle was to be elaborately decorated with fine twisted linen, blue, purple and scarlet yarn, with cherubim worked into tapestries by skilled craftsmen.

Gold and bronze would be everywhere. After the tabernacle was completed according to God's instructions, an amazing thing happened.

Then the cloud covered the Tent of Meeting, and the glory of the LORD filled the tabernacle (Exodus 40:34).

God had come to dwell among His people! Desiring intimacy and fellowship with His children, He displayed His power, majesty, and glory.

Another account of God's desire to be with His people can be found in the story of King Solomon's temple. His father, King David, had received instructions from God regarding all the specifications of the temple. Opulent in every way, there was a lavish use of the costliest of materials, including priceless amounts of gold and precious gems. Angels were woven into curtains of blue, purple, and crimson linen. The inner sanctuary was decorated with pure gold. The altar was overlaid with gold and above it were golden replicas of angels. The doors were made of wood with carved palm trees, open flowers, and angels, all overlaid with gold. It must have been an incredible sight. Solomon said, *The temple I am going to build will be great, because our God is greater than all other gods* (2 Chronicles 2:5). The wonderful drama continues seven years later as Solomon leads the people in the dedication of the completed temple. Before they can complete the ceremony, history is again repeated:

When the priests withdrew from the Holy Place, the cloud filled the temple of the LORD. And the priests could not perform their service because of the cloud, for the glory of the LORD filled his temple (I Kings 8:10–11).

Again God showed up on the scene displaying His glory and wonder. It was so stunning, in fact, that the priests could not continue the service. In his prayer, Solomon makes a powerful declaration,

But will God really dwell on earth? The heavens, even the highest heaven, cannot contain you. How much less this temple I have built! (1 Kings 8:27)

Solomon's magnificent monument to our God no longer exists. It was destroyed when His people were taken into exile, years before the birth of Christ. Ezra later oversaw the rebuilding of the temple, and Herod enhanced the visible grandeur of that structure. However, it, too, was destroyed by the Romans in A.D. 70. Today, rather than residing in a building, God has chosen instead to dwell in the hearts, lives, souls, and *bodies* of men and women. This is the way He is made known to others, as Paul wrote, *Christ in you, the hope of glory* (Colossians 1:27). God is our foundation (Isaiah 33:6) and our body is His temple (1 Corinthians 6:19). We have the profound privilege of welcoming the presence of God to dwell within us, just as He once dwelt within Moses' tabernacle and Solomon's temple.

The dwelling places He chose for His glory were extravagant in every detail. Likewise our bodies are very special to God because He is the master architect, the landlord, and He has chosen to join us in tenancy. God doesn't dwell in the mediocre. He chooses only the most splendid structures in which to live.

Are you beginning to catch a glimpse of just how incredible and special you are in God's eyes? God esteems you. You are a favored one. You are an expression of His glory, created in His image to know Him personally and to make Him known.

As we continue this journey, let's remember that we are in the process of rebuilding or restoring the temple in which He has chosen to dwell. Thankfully we don't have to wait until the work in us is completed before He comes to live in us. His work on the cross is completed, and because of that He chooses to dwell within us now. Let's be certain that our bodies, as His temples are suitable for His indwelling presence.

With these things in mind, you can honor and trust your body more completely when it comes to food and eating. Continue to build with the finest materials. Anything artificial or lacking authenticity would not be His desire. Can you imagine a temple overlaid with fool's gold? We want to be certain that every stone and cedar beam we offer God is solidly laid on the love He has for us.

At the king's command they removed from the quarry large blocks of quality stone to provide a foundation of dressed stone for the temple. The craftsmen . . . cut and prepared the timber and stone for the building of the temple (1 Kings 5:17–18).

Let's turn our attention to some contemplative introspection. Consider what follows to be part of your own personal "cutting and preparing process," the work God is doing in you, His temple. Anything that pushes us toward eating when we aren't hungry, when we're not yet at that empty 0 runs counter to our godly goals. On Day Two John, after having breakfast, began eating donuts when he wasn't hungry. We call this unconscious behavior "fat machinery." Have you noticed yourself doing similar things?

You may be becoming more aware of this behavior if you are taking bodometer readings this week.

As technical as this may sound, you will discover that it is quite illuminating to identify what in your life acts as fat machinery, turning you to food when you aren't yet at 0.

Fat Machinery

What causes you to turn to food when you are not hungry? When we follow the inclinations of our flesh our fat machinery usually falls into one or more of four different categories. We highlight each now, but we'll investigate the categories separately in the days to come.

1. Conditioned or habitual responses. These are thoughts or actions that cause our "eat button" to be pressed; for instance, eating while watching TV. If we do this often enough, we will come to a place where we end up eating every time the TV goes on, whether or not we're hungry.

2. Beliefs. Some of us were taught that we need three "square" meals each day in order to be healthy. This may be appropriate for people who have strenuous jobs, but thinking that it applies to everyone is inaccurate. There was a time when I paid no attention to my body's requirements and I ate like a hired hand even though I was doing sedentary work. Beliefs such as this interfere with giving our bodies just the nourishment they need, only when they need it. Today I enjoy eating when I am truly hungry, which may be once a day or three times a day.

3. Past Stories. These include the experiences and situations that have influenced your eating and weight problems. Laurie serves as a good example. She had a very traumatic experience that triggered obsessive eating for twenty-seven years. After being raped and assaulted by her boyfriend, her mother refused to speak to her except to call her names. Laurie eventually began to believe that every word her mother said about her was true.

Laurie explains, "I gained thirty pounds within a few months and have struggled with gaining even more weight ever since. I used food as comfort and a means of escape. Food became my god. I started on a self-destructive path because I felt used and worthless, and I believed it had been my fault. I kept the secret for twenty-seven years, and it ate at me every day as my weight continued to escalate."

Now that Laurie has looked more carefully at her past, she sees that she can dismantle the beliefs that have resulted in fat machinery eating. In this process and with God's help, she has released fifty pounds.

4. Failures. Most people have had problems trying to lose weight with diets. Diets deal with symptoms and never with the real causes of eating when we aren't hungry. By using the Thin Within tools and depending on the leading of the Spirit within, you can observe the causes of your unworkable eating habits and the origins of your fat machinery. It is important that you understand what makes you tick. You can then observe and correct, making adjustments that take you closer to your godly goal of being conformed to the image of Christ from the inside out.

One example of fat machinery in action is our reliance on, and our response to, the bathroom scale. Consider your use of the scale over the years. How has it served you? Has it helped you reach or remain at your desired size? Or has it been used to justify overeating? How often do you jump on a scale? Once a week? Five times a day?

Most of us can relate to one of three scenarios: First, you hop on the scale and it says you have gained weight. Depressed, you go to the kitchen and drown your sorrows in a megabreakfast. Second, you hop on the scale and it says you have lost weight. You are so excited you celebrate by eating a hot fudge sundae. In the third scenario you avoid the scale like the plague because you know very well that your weight is creeping up and you don't want to face the awful truth. Has your scale become a club of condemnation? Is it an idol? Does your bathroom scale determine whether you have a good day or a bad day?

We would like to encourage you to put the scale in its proper place, maybe in the closet or garage where you won't be tempted to misuse it and also so that it won't control your life. We often think things are better or worse than they actually are, so prayerfully using the scales as a reality check from time to time is OK. However, we don't want the scales to become an idol. In order to avoid that, we strongly suggest that you replace the man-made bathroom scales with the daily use of your God-given hunger scale and 0 to 5 eating.

How will you know if you are releasing weight? As you dress you will see and feel the difference: your belt will become looser and your pants not so tight. Trust your body and trust God. He will lead you to your natural size.

One of our participants named Olivia said, "Part of the program involved putting away the scale, but I brought mine back out after it had lost its power over me. It's now a friend, and I don't let it affect how I eat."

Take Action

+ Continue to persevere in your commitment to eat between 0 and 5.
+ Today we have exposed some of the challenges you may face in using the first Key to Conscious Eating—eating only when you are hungry. We will investigate each of these four categories in more depth in the days to come. Now we offer you a practical tool to assist in observing and correcting. It is called the Thin Within Food Log. It is a visual aid that can be very helpful on your journey through our next twenty-four days.

Thin Within Food Log

Hunger # Before Eating	Time	Items/Amount	Hunger # After Eating
0	Noon	Peanuts (handful)	3

It bears repeating—this is a grace-based process. If at any time during these thirty days you feel led to stop using any of these tools, feel free to do so. For now, however, you might want to utilize this one. It is not like any other food log in that you don't need to weigh and measure, count calories or fat grams. All you need to do is jot down your hunger level, the time, what you ate, the approximate amount, and your hunger level after you ate.

In doing so, you'll see what barriers to conscious eating are standing in your way. It is a wonderful opportunity to observe your own behavior and then to apply the correction that will line up your behavior with your goal of 0 to 5 eating.

Your Success Story

Did you have any new insights while you were reading today? Please record them below.

_____

_____

_____

Verses to Ponder

No distrust made him waiver concerning the promise of God, but he grew strong in his faith as he gave glory to God, being fully convinced that God was able to do what he had promised. Therefore his faith was reckoned to him as righteousness (Romans 4:20–22, NRSV).

Now devote your heart and soul to seeking the LORD *your God. Begin to build the sanctuary of the* LORD *God* (1 Chronicles 22:19a).

Prayer

Thank You, Lord, that You have made my body the temple of Your Holy Spirit. Thank You for choosing to live within me. I am honored and I welcome You to do Your work in me from the inside out. I pray that You will help me to recognize true stomach hunger. Help me to listen to and trust the signals that my body sends me. When I am in doubt, help me to pause and ask You for strength and guidance. Thank You that You are with me to guide me on this journey. In Jesus' name, Amen.

Medical Moment

Physical hunger involves a complicated interaction between the brain, the endocrine system, and the digestive system. Much of it is not completely understood. We do know that the brain receives the message that signals hunger from the stomach, the upper intestinal tract, the liver, and from our fat stores. However, these true signals that the body needs nourishment are often overshadowed by emotions or external stimuli that can result in inappropriate eating. A little-appreciated fact is how small an amount of food is required to satisfy our hunger (your mother was correct when she said that you wouldn't want dinner if you ate that after-school snack.) The stomach is hugely distensible, as witnessed to by the prodigious quantities of food that can be consumed at a single sitting, but a feeling of comfort can be achieved by much less food than you might imagine. (Try eating just half of an ordinary meal and you'll see.) A peculiarity of our digestive system is that it takes about twenty minutes for our brain to register how full we are, which means it's possible to continue eating for twenty minutes beyond a point of comfort. That explains the discomfort we feel by stuffing ourselves at Thanksgiving or other times when we eat large quantities rather quickly.

—ARTHUR HALLIDAY, M.D.

Success Tools
+ Wait until you are at a 0 before eating.
+ Fill in the Thin Within Food Log.
+ Use the Thin Within Observations and Corrections Chart today.
+ Use the Thin Within Keys to Conscious Eating when you choose to eat or drink today.

Thin Within Food Log

Hunger # before Eating	Time	Items/Amount	Hunger # after Eating

Thin Within Observations and Corrections Chart—Day 6

Observations	Day 6
1. I ate when my body was hungry.	
2. I ate in a calm environment by reducing distractions.	
3. I ate when I was sitting.	
4. I ate when my body and mind were relaxed.	
5. I ate and drank the things my body enjoyed.	
6. I paid attention to my food while eating.	
7. I ate slowly, savoring each bite.	
8. I stopped before my body was full.	

Thin Within Wisdom

Consider what could possibly happen if you wait for a 0? You might experience the joy of eating your meal when you are truly hungry!

My Body, God's Restoration Underway

*Trust in the LORD with all your heart
and lean not on your own understanding;
in all your ways acknowledge him,
and he will make your paths straight.*
—Proverbs 3:5–6

We have covered a lot of ground in a short time on our journey to freedom. We began by introducing the keys to conscious eating and the observation and correction tool, and pray that you are experiencing joy in eating this way. Remember God's grace is abundant, His forgiveness is forever freeing, and His love is never-ending.

If you stumble, go to God and let Him help you to observe, correct, and move on down the path of His provision. Above all, don't reach for the club of condemnation. As writer F. Scott Fitzgerald said, "Never confuse a single defeat with a final defeat." No defeat need be final. We will speak more to this issue on Day Ten.

Let's review for a minute by looking at figure 7-1. As we noted on Day Four, the person on the path of my performance is often lacking in confidence regarding God's love and acceptance. Although the person on this path may be a believer and under the canopy of grace, he isn't experiencing the ongoing full benefits of that grace. He suffers from a lack of faith that keeps him from moving forward. Caught between legalism and license, he never really makes progress. He moves from having an overflow of confidence in his own effort to being discouraged and feeling miserable.

The person on the path of God's provision, as we have seen, may experience a "two steps forward and one back" movement, but the direction is set. This person moves forward confident of God's love and acceptance through the cross of Christ. His or her life doesn't reflect an "on again-off again" experience, as the cross of Christ is a stabilizing force. His confidence is not in his own flesh, but in God's blessed provision. This person learns from her steps backward through observation and correction. No "failure" is beyond God's ability to redeem or His desire to make good. This person isn't perfect, by any means, but he or she moves forward trusting in God even after experiencing a setback.

Linda, a participant who released over eighty pounds, writes, "Weight loss is a small part of the wonderful benefits of Thin Within. Learning from my failures helps me live in the present time and enjoy each and every day."

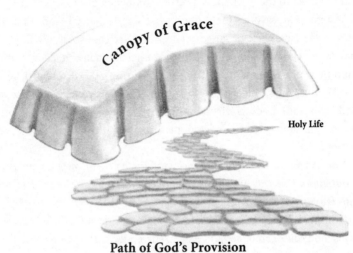

Path of God's Provision
Two Steps Forward and One Back • Leading Toward the Holy Life • Confidence in God

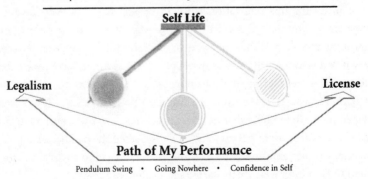

Path of My Performance
Pendulum Swing   •   Going Nowhere   •   Confidence in Self

figure 7–1

By now you have seen the value of becoming more intentional about your eating, what we call "eating in present time." We hope that you are rejoicing in the newfound freedom you have from diet laws, diet rules, and diet foods. Now you can enjoy any food with 0 to 5 eating, using your God-given internal hunger scale.

You have also looked at God's goals and His vision for you. He wants so much for you to experience the fullness of His plan by aligning your goals and vision with His plans for you. On Day Three, you set some godly goals for our thirty days together, keeping your eyes on the purpose for which you were created. God created you to glorify Him, to make Him known, and to reflect to the world how awesome and wonderful He is.

Yesterday we savored the thought that we are indeed God's incredible temple, the tabernacle or sanctuary in which He chooses to dwell. But you may have begun this journey after encountering many challenges in your life, and by now you may feel like a temple in ruins. Be encouraged, because as A.W. Tozer says, you are "glorious ruins." Perhaps you feel that honoring God with your body is virtually impossible because you think you are beyond His ability to repair, let alone to indwell. If so, God has a promise for you:

Your people will rebuild the ancient ruins and will raise up the age-old foundations; you will be called Repairer of Broken Walls, Restorer of Streets with Dwellings (Isaiah 58:12).

Nothing is beyond the reach of His restoration project. Even ancient and devastated ruins can be rebuilt. As you surrender to the Master Builder you will be His apprentice repairer and restorer.

In order for this renovation work to be effective, however, we must understand why the ruins exist. It is important for us to investigate our emotions and the part they may play in our eating. This is especially necessary if you view your life as a heap of rubble. God longs to take your tribulation and redeem it for wondrous purposes.

Barbara, who released over one hundred pounds, says, "Thin Within helped me to figure out whether I was eating because I was hungry, out of rebellion, or for emotional reasons." She discovered she had been suppressing many of her emotions, and as those feelings began to surface, she took them to God in prayer which started her healing process.

When you look at the rubble of your life, you may not feel that you are equipped to deal with the devastation of your past or strong enough to face the task ahead. You may even see yourself as your own worst enemy. In fact, you may feel, at times, like the people of Judah:

Meanwhile, the people in Judah said, "The strength of the laborers is giving out, and there is so much rubble that we cannot rebuild the wall" (Nehemiah 4:10).

Be encouraged. Our Lord will meet you and enable you. Invite Him to help you to clear away the rubble on your path. The rebuilding process goes much more smoothly when the way is adequately prepared. He longs to do this with you. We prayerfully ask you to persevere, knowing that God's gentle, guiding hand will strengthen you.

So do not fear, for I am with you; do not be dismayed, for I am your God. I will strengthen you and help you; I will uphold you with my righteous right hand (Isaiah 41:10).

Ralph Waldo Emerson has said, "We do not believe there is any force today to rival or recreate that beautiful yesterday. We linger in the ruins of the old tent, where once we had bread and shelter, nor believe that the spirit can feed, cover, and nerve us again. We cannot again find aught so dear, so sweet, so graceful. But we sit and weep in vain. The voice of the Almighty saith, 'Up and onward for evermore.' We cannot stay amid the ruins."[1]

With that in mind, let's refuse to stay amid the ruins and move onward. There is great hope and freedom ahead.

Take Action

+ Today you will become more aware of feelings and experiences that may lure you to eat when you aren't yet empty. You may want to recommit to eating only when you are hungry and diligently apply yourself to using the Keys to Conscious Eating.

Emotional Eating Exercise

Pray first to experience God's comfort, strength, and help. Trust that He will uphold you as you complete Exercise 7-1. Look at the situations or states of mind in the left-hand column. Consider the first one and imagine that you are angry. Close your eyes and recall a time when you were angry. What food or drink comes to mind when you envision yourself feeling angry? Perhaps your answer is pretzels. Then ask yourself: How do I eat pretzels when I'm angry? One at a time? A whole handful at once while pacing back and forth? Or perhaps you quickly shove them into your mouth while standing in the kitchen or watching TV. Whatever your response, write it down in the appropriate column.

In order to receive the greatest benefit through this process, don't analyze to see if your answer is "correct." Just record what comes to mind as you picture yourself experiencing each emotion. The same food or drink may come to mind more than once. As you do this, simply observe and refrain from self-condemnation. Remember, there is no condemnation for those who are in Christ Jesus.

Exercise 7-1 Emotional Eating Exercise

Situation or State of Mind	Food or Drink	Manner of Eating
Angry	Pretzels	Standing in the kitchen stuffing mindlessly while slamming the cupboard doors.
Bored		
Overwhelmed		
Tired		
Sick		
Depressed		
Tense, anxious		
Frustrated		
Lonely, unloved		
Unexpressed anger		
Self-hate, disgust		
Guilt		
Procrastinating		
Indecision		
Feeling Insecure		

Busy		
Excited		
Having Fun		
Reward		
Luxuriousness		
Feeling secure		
Family holidays		
Remembering Mother		
Remembering Father		
Remembering any important figure in your life		

✦ Review what you have written. Do you notice any patterns or repetitive behavior? Prayerfully take to God what you have observed in your chart. Ask Him to help you face what you've discovered with honesty and a commitment to change.

_____

_____

_____

✦ Now we will offer an extended list of reasons that trigger inappropriate eating patterns.

Circle those that apply to you:

Reasons We Overeat

Worry-wart eating
Preventive eating (I might get hungry later so I'll eat now)
Nervous nibbling
Tourist eating (it may be my last chance to have an exotic eclair)

Eating because it's there, and I want it now

Eating out of happiness, sadness, etc.

Pleasing-the-hostess eating

Note that all of these responses come from our fat machinery rather than our body's hunger messages. It is a way we respond without heeding the voice of the Spirit. We merely react. Why do we eat like this? Here are some reasons that cause us to choose to eat when we aren't hungry:

"I get weak if I don't eat three meals a day."

"I have to attend too many business lunches."

"I come from a family of big eaters."

"I've always been heavy."

"Everyone in my family is overweight."

"I could never stop eating just one scoop of ice cream."

"I have to attend too many social events."

"I am just big boned."

"I need to reward myself."

"When I am stressed, food makes me feel good."

Each of these reasons, if allowed to go unchallenged, acts as a termite-infested cedar beam in God's temple. You would never want to build with materials that weren't what they appear to be on the outside. Eating for such reasons will not uphold your desire to reflect God's design for your natural size. We must work with our Lord to release any "building blocks" that aren't made of the purest truth in Christ. Let's get rid of second-rate building materials that will not support His temple.

Turning Off Your Fat Machinery

Because you want to restore your temple with authentic, quality materials, you must eradicate any false beliefs that perpetuate your fat machinery. The next time you get upset and head for the refrigerator, knowing you're not at 0, ask yourself these three questions:

1. Am I really hungry?

2. What is my hunger number right now?

3. Do I want to "stuff" my feelings by eating?

+ Wouldn't it be better to take your unmet needs, emotions, and will-fulness to the Lord in prayer? Asking these questions can help you to experience progress as you head down this road of restoration. At times your emotions may rage and seem absolutely uncontrollable. If so, take a moment to pray, asking God to help you respond in a way that honors your body and brings Him glory.

Fat Machinery Log

Below, record any of your personal fat machinery ("I paid for it so I should eat all of it"), from others ("You have to clean your plate"), and from the media ("Feed the Need"). As you observe and correct your fat machinery you will be amazed at the changes that will occur in your eating patterns.

Fat Machinery in Me	Fat Machinery from Others	Fat Machinery from Media

+ It can be a very enlightening experience to keep a log of your fat machinery as it rears its ugly head. As you do this, you will become aware of how fat machinery subtly filters into media, advertisements, conversations, and thoughts. Maybe you find yourself going to and from the kitchen looking for something to eat. Maybe your car automatically seems to stop at your favorite ice-cream parlor every time you try to drive by. Maybe thoughts of certain people make you want to eat (for instance, when Thomas thinks of his friend, Ben, he thinks of pizza.). Write down each experience as it occurs. Then ask yourself what that incident has to do with 0 to 5 eating. The answer is nothing.

+ If you are truly hungry, determine what would best satisfy you and then eat or drink that to a comfortable 5 or less on the hunger scale.

+ To uncover your fat machinery and switch it off, you can put up a few signs on the refrigerator or cupboard to interrupt your unconscious responses. Signs like "Am I really hungry?" or "Do I want to bury my feelings by eating when I'm not hungry?" or "Do I really want to be my natural God-given size?"

✦ As you become more aware of your fat machinery you will have a wonderful opportunity to grow in your dependence on the Lord. Consciously call upon Him and ask specifically what He would have you do to respond rather that react. Remember the observation and correction tool? This is a great time to apply it. Relish your increasing dependence on the Lord as He continues to lead you on this road to freedom.

Your Success Story

Did you have any new insights while you were reading today? Please record them below.

_____

_____

_____

Verses to Ponder

For no one can lay any foundation other than the one already laid, which is Jesus Christ (1 Corinthians 3:11).

I pray that out of his glorious riches he may strengthen you with power through his Spirit in your inner being, so that Christ may dwell in your hearts through faith (Ephesians 3:16–17a).

I can do everything through him who gives me strength (Philippians 4:13).

His divine power has given us everything we need for life and godliness through our knowledge of him who called us by his own glory and goodness (2 Peter 1:3).

Prayer

Dear God, at times I feel as if my life is a pile of rubble because of the many trials I have been through over the years and because of my own willful ways. Sometimes I don't see how You can possibly make me into anything remotely resembling an acceptable temple. I know now that the Bible says You have chosen to love me and live inside me. All I need to do is accept that truth. Help me to open my mind and my heart to You, and when I feel emotionally upset, Lord, help me turn to You rather than to food. In Jesus' name, Amen.

Medical Moment

There is an epidemic of diabetes in this country. Fifteen thousand new cases are diagnosed each year, a sixfold increase between 1958 and 2000. This increase is due almost entirely to Type 2 (what used to be called adult-onset) diabetes, which now—with its complications of heart attacks, strokes, kidney failure, and blindness—accounts for 190,000 deaths per year.

The good news is that Type 2 diabetes is always treatable and often preventable. Though there is a genetic predisposition to Type 2 diabetes, it is essentially always related to being overweight, which interferes with the action of insulin. There are four things that reduce elevated blood-sugar levels: eating less, reducing weight, exercise, and medication (pills or insulin injections). Very often Type 2 diabetes can be cured without drugs if the person reaches and maintains his/her natural God-given size and does some exercising several times a week.

Perseverance is the key to long-term success.

—ARTHUR HALLIDAY, M.D.

Success Tools

+ Use the Thin Within Food Log to continue to record hunger levels and what you eat today.
+ Use the Thin Within Observations and Corrections Chart today.
+ Use the Thin Within Keys to Conscious Eating when you choose to eat or drink today.

Thin Within Wisdom

Rather than condemn or reject, observe and correct. Refuse to condemn yourself, knowing that God loves you unconditionally.

NOTE
1.   Ralph Waldo Emerson.

Thin Within Food Log

Hunger # before Eating	Time	Items/Amount	Hunger # after Eating

Thin Within Observations and Corrections Chart—Day 7

Observations	Day 7
1. I ate when my body was hungry.	
2. I ate in a calm environment by reducing distractions.	
3. I ate when I was sitting.	
4. I ate when my body and mind were relaxed.	
5. I ate and drank the things my body enjoyed.	
6. I paid attention to my food while eating.	
7. I ate slowly, savoring each bite.	
8. I stopped before my body was full.	

Overcoming Obstacles to Restoration: Part 1

But as for you, be strong and do not give up,
for your work will be rewarded.
—2 Chronicles 15:7

What a blessing to know that God has promised that our hard work will be rewarded. His promises are true. He is faithful. He will strengthen us for the task set before us.

For the eyes of the LORD range throughout the earth to strengthen those whose hearts are fully committed to him (2 Chronicles 16:9a).

As we surrender our hearts fully to His Spirit, we continue now to build in the strength of the Lord. He knows our hearts. He wants to give us His strength and He doesn't expect us to succeed apart from Him.

The promise from 2 Chronicles 16:9a was first spoken to someone who had experienced the power of God when facing a great army that was marshaled against him. King Asa, one of Judah's kings after the reign of King Solomon, knew what it was like to see God fight the battle with and for him. With the outpouring of the almighty hand of God, a battle against all earthly odds was won. Today we too can apply the promise given to King Asa to our own lives and our Thin Within journey.

Asa had an exceptional beginning. He started strong. In fact, he was given one of the highest compliments ever paid to any king of Judah: *Asa did what was right in the eyes of the LORD, as his father David had done* (1 Kings 15:11). He jumped on the path of God's provision and committed himself to staying there.

Asa immediately got to work when he was put in charge of Judah. Pursuing a holy life, he rid the land of anything that didn't glorify God: *He brought into the temple of the LORD the silver and gold and the articles that he and his father had dedicated* (1 Kings 15:15). Asa esteemed the temple and began to adorn it in an appropriate manner, giving it the attention it deserved.

Perhaps, in a similar way, you have found yourself immediately applying the keys to conscious eating, using the observation and correction tool, and focusing yourself one hundred percent on this process. You are walking the path of God's provision and delighting in knowing that Christ is sufficient. We hope that you are already noticing some positive physical, emotional, and spiritual changes. You may even be experiencing a change in your attitude toward your body.

However, in Asa's case, just as things were going well, he was challenged. First, he experienced an assault to his faith that, much to his credit, he met with confidence and strength that only God can give. He asked God to defeat an overwhelming army that stood to attack Judah, and God answered (2 Chronicles 14).

We, too, may discover challenges along our new road to freedom. If so, we also can call upon the strength of God to help us, and He will. As we depend on Him, He will be faithful. *For the eyes of the LORD range throughout the earth to strengthen those whose hearts are fully committed to Him* (2 Chronicles 16:9).

Unfortunately, during another time of testing, Asa did not fare so well. When an enemy attacked him, Asa, in his fear, forgot about God. His emotions overruled his common sense. What did he do? He took all the silver and gold left in the treasuries of the Lord's temple and sent some of his men off with it to buy the help of another king, going against God's clear instructions prohibiting such an alliance.

Asa somehow thought that God's help wasn't enough (1 Kings 15:18–20). He forgot that God would provide him with everything he needed as He had done before. Asa sold out. He disregarded God and defiled His temple. In that moment of terror he believed the lie that his kingdom would be overtaken. This belief was at odds with deeper beliefs and values he previously had held. The belief that he needed a pagan king's help did not support his goal and vision of maintaining a holy kingdom set apart for the Lord. He had confidence in his own ability to work everything out the way he wanted which lead him down the path of his performance and away from God's best for him and his people.

What does Asa have to do with us? Just as he was sidetracked, any belief that results in eating when you're not hungry will not support your godly vision and goals to reach and maintain your natural God-given size. It will not help build the temple you are meant to be. If you haven't yet experienced such a challenge, scripture indicates that you soon will (James 1:2–4). There will be trials and temptations that come to us as we proceed along the road to freedom.

One participant confided: "It is a challenge to live consciously all the time rather than anesthetizing myself with food. When I'm anxious, I am still tempted to pop chocolate mints into my mouth instead of going to God. But I have discovered that if I don't stuff my feelings down with food, I am more sensitive to how the Lord is leading me."

We can decide in advance how we will respond to temptation. Will we cling to the truth of that which we hold most dear, or will we be controlled by beliefs that run counter to our deeper desires? God offers us the weaponry we need to face the enemy.

Therefore put on the full armor of God, so that when the day of evil comes, you may be able to stand your ground, and after you have done everything, to stand (Ephesians 6:13).

We don't need to allow unworkable beliefs to derail our godly vision and goals. We can put on the armor of God to defend the temple that He is restoring according to His plan and purpose.

One example of unworkable beliefs relates to hypoglycemia, or low blood sugar. Lillian, a Thin Within participant, complained that she was unable to lose weight because her doctor insisted that she eat six meals a day to maintain normal blood-sugar levels. Yet by using the Thin Within tools and eating only two small meals a day, plus a little snack at other times as her doctor instructed, she released twenty-two pounds by the end of the program. Lillian was ecstatic, as was her doctor. Naturally if you have a health problem of any kind, it is important to consult with your physician before making any changes in your eating.

One of the first things you will want to do is identify those unworkable beliefs that may be present in your mind. Once you have recognized them, you can subject them to the most powerful of weapons.

For though we live in the world, we do not wage war as the world does. The weapons we fight with are not the weapons of the world. On the contrary, they have divine power to demolish strongholds. We demolish arguments and every pretension that sets itself up against the knowledge of God, and we take captive every thought to make it obedient to Christ (2 Corinthians 10:3–5).

Had King Asa demolished arguments and pretensions that were set up against God, he would have taken captive his fear. He would not have sought the help of an ungodly king and an ungodly nation. King Asa started out well but he ended badly, and there were consequences to this behavior (2 Chronicles 16:9b). We can learn from his mistakes. We can identify and take captive any unworkable beliefs that we have so they will no longer take us captive. Fear is a common area of attack. But we know the truth, which is that God's perfect love, activated by our faith, casts out fear.

In the space provided, make a list of all the beliefs about food, eating, and weight loss you have accumulated from television, teachers, books, doctors, newspapers, friends and family.

My Beliefs About Food, Eating, and My Weight

_____

_____

_____

Listed below are some beliefs that participants have shared. Do any of these ring true for you?

Never let myself get hungry.
Dieting is the only way to lose weight.
I have to clean my plate.
Chocolate makes me feel better.
Starch is fattening.
Once I eat one potato chip, I won't be able to stop.
I need caffeine to jumpstart my day.
Eat three square meals a day.
I always gain weight during the holidays.
Losing weight is so difficult.
People should like me, in spite of being overweight.
If I paid for it, I'll have to eat it.
If I refuse food, they'll think I don't like them.
I always gain weight back after I lose it.
If I lose weight, I'll be sickly.
I couldn't be thin forever.
I'm fat simply because I love food and like to eat.
The only way to lose weight is to stop eating.

Never skip a meal.

I was fat as a child so I'll be fat as an adult.

Fat means prosperity.

It's my metabolism.

I'm a compulsive overeater.

I'm a chocoholic.

Present-Time Eating

In considering your beliefs, do you see any contradictions? (Example: I have to start my day with a cup of coffee, but coffee gives me an acid stomach.) Which beliefs have worked against you and which have supported you? Unworkable beliefs can be very powerful. They may, however, be so subtle that we accept them as facts rather than recognizing them as false beliefs or lies.

If King Asa had realized this as he was heading for the temple treasury to steal the silver and gold, he would have asked himself, "Are there any contradictions here? Hmm. I want to have a kingdom that honors God yet now I am taking all of the silver and gold to a pagan king because I am afraid that the impending battle is too great for God to win." If he had realized the folly of his thinking, perhaps he would have remained faithful to the Lord and to the temple that had been entrusted to his care.

Evaluate your beliefs at this point. Place them under godly, prayerful scrutiny to determine where they came from. At one time I believed I couldn't pass an ice-cream parlor without stopping and having several scoops. I had a reputation for being an ice-cream addict and I was determined to uphold my title! I now thank God I can enjoy ice cream on occasion. Instead of eating a whole quart, I have a satisfying amount of my favorite flavor and savor each bite.

A common belief that can lead to rationalizing is that any amount of weight gain is acceptable during pregnancy, despite abundant medical evidence to the contrary. To apply the Thin Within Keys to Conscious Eating during this special time might seem inappropriate, but we have had many women use the Thin Within tools when they were pregnant. We have found that 0 to 5 eating uniformly results in less weight gain, fewer blood pressure and diabetes problems, more comfortable and enjoyable pregnancies, and happier mothers, babies, and obstetricians. What a wonderful time to honor your body, God's temple.

Making Choices

King Asa could have evaluated other possibilities for his predicament. He wasn't backed up against a wall, as he feared. He could have asked himself, "Besides selling out, what other options do I have?" Likewise, the next time you're headed for that favorite ice-cream shop, ask yourself about other options. In fact, let's review the three questions we introduced yesterday, and add a fourth one. These are the questions you can ask yourself whenever you notice your fat machinery kicking in.

1. Am I really hungry?
2. What is my hunger number right now?
3. Do I want to "stuff" my feelings by eating?
4. What other options do I have besides eating?

What could you choose to do that would serve you better than eating when you are not truly hungry? You can turn to God in prayer, go for a walk, read, go to a movie, call a friend, clean out your closet, write a letter, pick flowers, read your Bible, take a nap. The list is endless.

List some creative options you could consider:

_____

_____

_____

Preplanning for Trials

We can preplan options before we are backed into a corner. If King Asa had prepared a contingency "battle plan" in case of an enemy attack, he would have more likely set aside any false beliefs, maintained his resolve, and avoided his downfall. Consider situations that can cause you to turn to food. Does it happen when the kids come home from school? When the stock market is down? When you face a deadline at work? By anticipating potential challenges, you can be prepared for the battle.

Take Action

+ Take stock of the stressors in your life. In the chart below, identify situations that you may face in the future. For each, identify the emotion or unworkable belief that may result from the situation. In the third column, record a strategy that will honor your body instead of compromising your values (see example).

✦ As with all the exercises in this book, we encourage you to pray before you begin, asking for godly wisdom.

Sometimes, of course, you won't see challenges coming and you will have to ask yourself on the spot, "What is really important to me? Are there any thoughts I need to take captive? What are my godly options?" Answering these questions will help you make wise choices.

Planning for Trials Exercise

Stressful Situation	Emotions that Can Trigger Inappropriate Eating	Appropriate Godly Strategy
Mother in-law coming to visit	Anxiety; Inadequacy; Feelings of being judged	Before she arrives, I will pray. Also, while she is here, I will journal before I eat.

Our God is a God of second, third, and umpteen chances. No matter how many times we may stumble, if we turn in humble dependence to Him, He will allow us to regain our forward momentum and continue with His restoration work. Remember the process of observation and correction. Even though Asa faltered as a ruler and steward of God's temple, he is honored in 1 Kings 15:14: *Asa's heart was fully committed to the LORD all his life.* He must have observed and corrected. Overcoming the obstacles of unworkable beliefs is an essential element in our walk with God. With the Holy Spirit as our ever-present guide, we, too, will continue making progress forward on the path of God's provision.

Your Success Story

Did you have any new feelings or ideas while you were reading today?
Please record them.

_____

_____

_____

Verses to Ponder

Therefore, my dear brothers, stand firm. Let nothing move you. Always give
yourselves fully to the work of the Lord, because you know that your labor in
the Lord is not in vain (1 Corinthians 15:58).

Therefore we do not lose heart. Though outwardly we are wasting away, yet
inwardly we are being renewed day by day. For our light and momentary trou-
bles are achieving for us an eternal glory that far outweighs them all. So we fix
our eyes not on what is seen, but on what is unseen. For what is seen is tem-
porary, but what is unseen is eternal (2 Corinthians 4:16–18).

Prayer

Dear Lord, there have been times when I have struggled to hang in there
and remain strong. Help me to keep my eyes focused on You and the goal
ahead. Help me to identify and deal with any unworkable beliefs, circum-
stances, or rebelliousness in me that can trigger my fat machinery. I want
to continue to follow You all the days of my life. In Jesus' name, Amen.

Medical Moment

Emotions truly are connected with our eating. The entire digestive system is under the direct control of the brain, starting with the smells of food
that are processed by a portion of the brain that also deals with emotions
and memory. This accounts for much of the psychology so strongly connected with eating—like memories of your mother's apple pies. Understanding this and dealing with your emotions from a godly perspective
will assist you on the path to freedom.

—Arthur Halliday, M.D.

Success Tools

+ Review your list of creative options in the Planning for Trials Exercise and put them into practice.
+ Keep adding to your Fat Machinery Log.
+ Continue to keep your food log, checking your hunger numbers before and after you eat.
+ Use your Thin Within Observations and Corrections Chart for today.
+ Use the Thin Within Keys to Conscious Eating.

Thin Within Food Log

Hunger # before Eating	Time	Items/Amount	Hunger # after Eating

Thin Within Observations and Corrections Chart—Day 8

Observations	Day 8
1. I ate when my body was hungry.	
2. I ate in a calm environment by reducing distractions.	
3. I ate when I was sitting.	
4. I ate when my body and mind were relaxed.	
5. I ate and drank the things my body enjoyed.	
6. I paid attention to my food while eating.	
7. I ate slowly, savoring each bite.	
8. I stopped before my body was full.	

Thin Within Wisdom

If you are not hungry, and you want to eat, your soul is crying out to meet with God. Go to Him in prayer.

Overcoming Obstacles to Restoration: Part 2

. . . and provide for those who grieve in Zion—
to bestow on them a crown of beauty instead of ashes,
the oil of gladness instead of mourning,
and a garment of praise instead of a spirit of despair.
They will be called oaks of righteousness,
a planting of the LORD for the display of his splendor.
—Isaiah 61:3

Isn't it wonderful to rest in the assurance that our God will supply all of our needs? The path of God's provision offers rest and peace as we trust in Him.

Yesterday we focused on how we often respond to emotions by eating our way through them. In moments such as these, we have a power greater than ourselves upon which to draw. We did some preplanning for some potential trials in our lives so we can have a way of escape other than through the cookie jar.

God's grace is an amazing gift, and His pardon is a priceless treasure. But that is not all. His presence always accompanies us and His power is available to implement whatever He calls us to do. Further, God's grace is an ongoing provision, providing insight, wisdom, and discernment as we continue down His path toward the holy life.

This path is full of adventure. As with any adventure you may discover the terrain is not always smooth. When the Lord Jesus made the great exchange upon the cross, he traded our ashes for His beauty, our mourning for His gladness, our despair for His praise. What an incredible legacy He left, giving each of us a crown of beauty, the oil of gladness, and garments of praise to adorn our temple. These are all ours as we allow Him to continue the work He has begun.

[Be] confident of this, that he who began a good work in you will carry it on to completion until the day of Christ Jesus (Philippians 1:6).

He will complete the work. He is God. He is king. As we allow His work to proceed, long-standing blockades and strongholds will begin to collapse. Obstacles that no earthly strength can remove will be reduced to dust by the power of the Holy Spirit.

God can take our troubles and use them to accomplish His purposes in our lives. This transformation process, this metamorphosis from ashes to beauty, is seen throughout the pages of Scripture. Of course, the most obvious example is the death of our Lord and Savior Jesus Christ upon the cross. When death thought it had dealt its final blow to the Son of God, His resurrection power reigned victorious instead.

Where, O death, is your victory? Where, O death, is your sting? (1 Corinthians 15:55)

David as a lowly shepherd learned to trust the Lord in destroying the lion and the bear. He discovered a strength beyond his own to fight off wild animals, destroy Goliath, and develop survival skills in the wild while running from a madman. God used all these challenges to form His shepherd for His sheep, Israel. David was a man after God's own heart—a warrior, a shepherd, a singer, and a poet. But he didn't start out as a hero. He was considered the least desirable son, the least likely to succeed. All of the trials of his lowly shepherd days formed his character for the ruling of God's chosen nation. Do you identify with David as the least likely to succeed? If so, be encouraged because you are exactly who God chooses to use for His purposes.

God's word contains innumerable examples of His power to transform lives. Paul's imprisonments were used to spread the gospel even to Caesar's household (Philippians 4:22). The persecution of the Christians caused the church to explode with growth (Acts 8:4). The shame of a promiscuous woman led her to draw water from a well where an encounter with the Savior satisfied her spiritual thirst with living water (John 4:6–7). Our God is in the business of taking straw and spinning it to gold! He truly does take our ashes and by applying His immeasurable grace turns them to a crown of beauty. He takes our mourning and turns them to garments of praise. He takes our broken lives and makes them a planting to display His splendor! *What good will it be for a man if he gains the whole world, yet forfeits his soul?* (Matthew 16:26a)

It is often true that a person will lose the world and yet gain his or her soul for eternity. When Thin Within was in a state of financial bankruptcy back in the 1980s, it felt as if my whole world was collapsing. This traumatic experience demonstrated the spiritual bankruptcy of my own soul. God used it to give me new life in Him. He redeemed my failures and went about rebuilding Thin Within on His word for His eternal purposes. We can't know the ways of God, which are beyond our comprehension. We can only turn to Him and, along with Job, say:

Though he slay me, yet will I hope in him (Job 13:15a).

If you ask me now if I would rather have Thin Within in its early years of solid financial standing or the crisis that brought me to Christ, the answer would be crystal clear. I want Him. I count anything else as rubbish so that I can gain Christ (Philippians 3:7–8). Are we minimizing the pain and suffering of life itself? Not at all. We merely emphasize the fact that our current suffering isn't the only truth upon which to focus. It isn't even the *primary* truth. What our sovereign God has purposed in Heaven is more real than what we can see.

Therefore we do not lose heart. Though outwardly we are wasting away, yet inwardly we are being renewed day by day. For our light and momentary troubles are achieving for us an eternal glory that far outweighs them all. So we fix our eyes not on what is seen, but on what is unseen. For what is seen is temporary, but what is unseen is eternal (2 Corinthians 4:16–18).

We can't begin to fathom the ways of God. His ways are not our ways and His thoughts are not our thoughts (Isaiah 55:8). There is no way to prove that He is justified in what He does. The fact of the matter is God is God. He needs no justification. In the words of author Brennan Manning, "He is not moody or capricious; He knows no seasons of change. He has a single relentless stance toward us. He loves us."[1]

We can rest assured that no suffering is wasted when it is placed in God's hands. No single heart aches that His doesn't ache all the more. The Scriptures teach that the Lord has a record of all our tears (Psalm 56:8). We know that Jesus wept with Mary and Martha at the death of their brother, Lazarus (John 11:35). We know that one day our Lord will wipe away every tear from our eyes (Revelation 7:17).

God uses each and every tear we have shed and every pain we have experienced to form and mold our character, to strengthen us, and to draw us closer to His heart. He wants us to experience His strength and sufficiency. He uses affliction to cause us to see our need for Him and our struggles with food, eating, and our bodies to send us to Him, to look for *His* solution. In our weakness, He is made strong. He uses even this personal battle you are experiencing and He will redeem it for His glory.

The psalmist wrote, *Before I was afflicted I went astray, but now I obey your word. You are good, and what you do is good* (Psalm 119:67–68).

Joni Eareckson Tada, who had a diving accident as a youth that resulted in her becoming a paraplegic, encourages us in her book *When God Weeps*:

"Before my paralysis, my hands reached for a lot of wrong things and my feet took me into some bad places. After my paralysis, tempting choices were scaled down considerably.

"God uses suffering to purge sin from our lives, strengthen our commitment to Him, force us to depend on grace, bind us together with other believers, produce discernment, foster sensitivity, discipline our minds, spend our time wisely, stretch our hope, cause us to know Christ better, make us long for truth, lead us to repentance of sin, teach us to give thanks in times of sorrow, increase faith, and strengthen character. It is a beautiful image."[2]

This woman of God said she used to pray, "God just get me out of this wheelchair." Today she says, "If it weren't for this wheelchair I wouldn't be used of God as I am today." She gives glory to God for His purpose and plans. What a great perspective she has. We too can be sure that whatever life brings will be used of God to harmonize with His plan and purpose for us. His intention is not to harm us but to help us prosper and to give us hope and a future (Jeremiah 29:11). It may not be in this life that we realize the full reality of this hope and future. It may be in eternity.

As we choose to believe that He turns our trials into something beneficial for our growth, we can experience in a fresh way just how good He is. We grow in the Spirit when we begin to understand His sovereignty and His loving nature in all things. There is security in trusting Him, in believing that He and His purposes are good. We can rest in Him, confident in His love that will see us through the difficulties that challenge us.

Anita, a participant who released twenty pounds, said, "Through Thin Within I came to see that the trials I had faced and the way I had chosen to deal with them—by running to food—were actually God's way of calling me into closer fellowship with Him. When my food and eating problem became desperate, I saw my need for a great deliverer. God has taken my trials and hardships and used them to build my character and transform my life."

Through prayer, we can catch a glimpse of God's amazing purposes in our lives. Let's prayerfully investigate some of the ways He is conforming you to the image of Christ. He will not waste a single tear or a solitary heartache. He holds your future and longs to give you His hope.

Take Action

Evaluate some of the trials and challenging events that have happened in your life. Use the chart below to identify experiences that were hard for you. In the middle column record how you responded to the trial at the time. Did it cause you to question God's love? Did you get angry? Did you go into denial? Did you respond by eating your way through it? In the final column, recall anything positive that resulted from the experience. Here is an example for you.

Challenging Experience	How I responded at the time	Blessings that I can see that have come as a result of the trial
The financial collapse of Thin Within in the 1980s.	My life was in shambles and I thought my world was going to end.	Surrendered my life to Christ. Developed a thirst for God's Word. The transformation and restoration of Thin Within mirrored my own life change and God has used it to reflect His glory.

✦ Are you currently in the midst of a challenge or trial? If so, identify it in the space provided on page 90. Ask the Lord to reveal His purposes for allowing this trial and record what if anything He reveals to you. Conclude with a prayer that He will help you to believe that He is good and sovereign, even in the midst of this challenging time.

_____

_____

_____

✦ When you find yourself wanting to eat today, take a bodometer reading. Evaluate if you are at a 0 or if your desire to eat is triggered by emotions you are currently experiencing. Safeguard against allowing this time of reflection to send you to food. Instead, allow it to draw you nearer to the heart of God.

As the road that leads to freedom stretches before us, we need not turn aside from the bumps and the potholes. God's hand will be upon us as we continue to walk with Him, remembering that this road leads to liberty. The path of His glorious provision leads to the holy life in Christ. Each step is taken by faith and He has promised to cherish and protect us as we travel.

Your Success Story

Did you have any new feelings or ideas while you were reading today? Please record them.

_____

_____

_____

Verses to Ponder

Do you not know? Have you not heard? The LORD is the everlasting God, the Creator of the ends of the earth. He will not grow tired or weary, and his understanding no one can fathom (Isaiah 40:28).

Consider it pure joy, my brothers, whenever you face trials of many kinds, because you know that the testing of your faith develops perseverance. Perseverance must finish its work so that you may be mature and complete, not lacking anything (James 1:2–4).

Praise be to the God and Father of our Lord Jesus Christ. In his great mercy he has given us new birth into a living hope through the resurrection of Jesus Christ from the dead, and into an inheritance that can never perish, spoil or fade—kept in heaven for you, who through faith are shielded by God's power until the coming of the salvation that is ready to be revealed in the last time. In this you greatly rejoice, though now for a little while you may have had to suffer grief in all kinds of trials. These have come so that your faith—of greater worth than gold, which perishes even though refined by fire—may be proved genuine and may result in praise, glory and honor when Jesus Christ is revealed (1 Peter 1:3–7).

Medical Moment

Stress is challenging to define as it differs for each individual. One thing of which we can be sure, stress affects our physical, emotional, and spiritual health. If you find yourself in a situation of chronic stress, you might experience a variety of emotional or medical conditions such as eating disorders, depression, intestinal disorders, anxiety, insomnia, hypertension, and headaches. In addition, the general quality of your life can deteriorate. Because of this, we want to encourage you to deal with stress at its onset. Living a life of faith in an intimate relationship with the Lord can help tremendously. As we see things from God's perspective, we begin to take less and less of the worldly occurrences upon our own shoulders.

The power of prayer can truly have a tremendous impact in relieving stress as well. As we face issues that cause us concern, releasing them to the One who knows all things and is good, holy, and powerful, enables us to move on before we become "stressed out." As with most situations, God's word speaks to this issue directly. We are told in 1 Peter 5:7 to *cast all your anxiety on him because he cares for you.* Philippians 4:6–7 says, *Do not be anxious about anything, but in everything, by prayer and petition, with thanksgiving, present your requests to God. And the peace of God, which transcends all understanding, will guard your hearts and your minds in Christ Jesus.*

There is a peace that goes beyond our imaginings. It truly will be the most effective means to rid ourselves of stress and the medical conditions that accompany it.

—ARTHUR HALLIDAY, M.D.

Prayer

Dear Lord, please help me have faith that You are doing what is best. I want to believe that in all things You are good, and I pray that I will be able to rest in the assurance of Your love and Your sovereignty. Help me to mature and grow in my trust in You. I want to believe that You will take all the things that I face and work them out to be something beneficial. Help me to lean on You Lord, and not on my own understanding. In Your precious name I pray, Amen.

Success Tools

+ Continue to keep the Fat Machinery Log. This is your last day.
+ Continue to keep your food log with your hunger numbers.
+ Continue marking your Thin Within Observations and Corrections Chart.
+ Use the Thin Within Keys to Conscious Eating.

Thin Within Wisdom

Often what I see isn't all that my trials are about. I can take heart, knowing that God is about a bigger work.

Fat Machinery Log

Below, record any of your personal fat machinery ("I paid for it so I should eat all of it"), from others ("You have to clean your plate"), and from the media ("Feed the Need"). As you observe and correct your fat machinery you will be amazed at the changes that will occur in your eating patterns.

Fat Machinery in Me	Fat Machinery from Others	Fat Machinery from Media

Thin Within Food Log

Hunger # before Eating	Time	Items/Amount	Hunger # after Eating

Thin Within Observations and Corrections Chart—Day 9

Observations	Day 9
1. I ate when my body was hungry.	
2. I ate in a calm environment by reducing distractions.	
3. I ate when I was sitting.	
4. I ate when my body and mind were relaxed.	
5. I ate and drank the things my body enjoyed.	
6. I paid attention to my food while eating.	
7. I ate slowly, savoring each bite.	
8. I stopped before my body was full.	

NOTES

1. Brennan Manning, *The Ragamuffin Gospel* (Sisters, Oregon: Multnomah Books, 2000), 74.
2. Joni Eareckson Tada and Steve Estes, *When God Weeps—Why Our Sufferings Matter to the Almighty* (Grand Rapids, Michigan: Zondervan Publishing House, 1997), 117.

❧

Building in the Present Moment

Not that I have already obtained all this, or have already been made perfect,
but I press on to take hold of that for which Christ Jesus took hold of me.
Brothers, I do not consider myself yet to have taken hold of it.
But one thing I do: Forgetting what is behind
and straining toward what is ahead,
I press on toward the goal to win the prize for which God
has called me heavenwards in Christ Jesus.
—Philippians 3:12–14

"Press on!" What a powerful proclamation. What an inspiring challenge. When the battle is raging, when you are struggling, "press on." When you are enjoying the thrill of success and are tempted to camp there for a while, "press on."

Today, will you choose to "press on" rather than spend time reliving your defeats, or even your successes? Today, will you choose to continue to allow God to renew, restore, refresh, and remake you? He brings glorious wonder from what we think are defeats. He also equips us to sustain success. In each present moment, we can experience His joy, His abundance, and His grace afresh.

We are hard pressed on every side, but not crushed; perplexed, but not in despair; persecuted, but not abandoned; struck down, but not destroyed. We always carry around in our body the death of Jesus, so that the life of Jesus may also be revealed in our body (2 Corinthians 4:8–10).

Since we began our journey, have you been moving forward steadily, or have you been beating yourself up for your lack of success? Perhaps, if you are honest, you know that you've been eating between 3 and 7, not 0 and 5. If so, God's grace is sufficient. Maybe you haven't yet gotten past the temptation to binge. God's grace is still sufficient.

Please remember that God doesn't have plans to rake you over heavenly coals. His arms are always open. He longs to show you compassion as He calls you to follow Him. He is waiting for you, right here, right now. "Under grace we are free to turn to God as we really are, free to learn from our mistakes, free to change and grow, and free to allow Him to make us all he intends us to be."[1]

During the past nine days we have begun to see ourselves as God sees us. While it is true that we all fall short of His glory (Romans 3:23), He has also provided the solution to this dilemma (Romans 6:23). Because of the cross of Christ, God sees us as His beloved even when we feel like failures.

One Thin Within participant shared her new perspective on failure, "I've always been hard on myself, but now I've learned to move on. I'm on a journey through life. I'm *not* a failure, but a work in progress." Sheila, on the other hand, said, "I have always had a tendency to just give up when I would fail. I would let myself get so discouraged I would sink into self-pity that was sort of a permission to give into my own passive ways. It has been so helpful to see there is another path readily available."

If we see our "failures" through God's lens, we are much less likely to excuse our behavior or beat ourselves up over them. Through His eyes, perceived failures become opportunities. He sees our need and, in His grace, responds by coming alongside us to meet that need.

What is your reaction to a perceived failure? Do you sink under the weight of failure into defeat, or do you stand firm on the wisdom of failure? As Denis Waitley put it:

"Failure should be our teacher, not our undertaker. Failure is delay, not defeat. It is a temporary detour, not a dead end. Failure is something we can avoid only by saying nothing, doing nothing, and being nothing."[2]

Pastor Ray Johnston at Bayside Church in Granite Bay, California tells a story of the great pianist, Ignacy Jan Paderewski, who was to perform at Carnegie Hall. As the crowd waited politely for him to appear on stage, somehow a small child scampered up, climbed onto the piano bench, and proudly pounded out "Chopsticks" with his chubby little fingers. No mother or father was to be seen anywhere. The audience rustled uncomfortably, looking for someone to take care of this child who was disrupting the beginning of what was supposed to be a magnificent performance. Disapproving murmurs rose in volume and still no parents came forth. The little boy continued, delighting in the attention, oblivious to the whispers of displeasure.

Then the curtains parted and Paderewski himself appeared. The great musician approached the boy at the piano who remained unaware of his presence. Instead of scolding, ridiculing, or correcting the boy, the pianist placed his arms around him and began accompanying him in harmonious splendor. Never did "Chopsticks" get so fine a treatment or sound so beautiful.

Paderewski had the wisdom to discern that, rather than to scold or berate the child for his obvious faux pas, he could, instead, turn the child's "failure" into a masterpiece. Our Lord does the same and much more with our own strivings and failings. He sees the potential in our efforts, even when the results fall far short of our intention.

Why *do* we fail? Why are our best efforts lacking? Sometimes we fail because we leave God out of the equation. We think we know what is best in a situation or in terms of food choices, and we forget or neglect to consult the Great Physician, the one who spent great care in carefully crafting our bodies. This kind of failure can be accompanied by sin. If we go against God's precepts, we are called to turn to Him in confession and repentance. He is faithful and will cleanse us white as snow (Isaiah 1:18). A second reason we fail is we often try to act in our own strength. Rather than waiting on God and His timing, we run ahead of him. I don't know about you, but this is my area of weakness where I am tested time and again. I presume that God needs my help, when in truth He needs my humble dependence and patience as I wait on Him and Him alone. A third reason for failure is that we attempt a task to which we may not be called or gifted by God. Romans 12:3 reminds us not to think more highly of ourselves than we ought. It is important to recognize and readily admit our limitations as well as our strengths.

We are more apt to fail when we try to operate outside of our element. However, if we take each "failure" to God with the attitude of Benjamin Franklin, who said, "I haven't failed, I've found 10,000 things that don't work," we will discover just how much God can do. This is the wisdom that can come from our failure. When God's wisdom is applied, anything is possible.

Failure is not something we are. Failure is something we do. There is a big difference. When we take on the identity of "a failure," we begin to act more and more in keeping with that label. Labels can be debilitating. Instead we are to see ourselves as God sees us. Then we will begin to act in accordance with what He has already declared to be true.

Consider the following story: One day a naturalist was passing a farm. He glanced over at the chicken yard and noticed among the chickens pecking away at the corn one of the most beautiful eagles he had ever seen.

He said to the farmer, "What in the world is that eagle doing in the chicken pen?"

The farmer drawled, "Well, I really don't know, but he seems to think he's a chicken. He's been there for a long time and he won't leave. I've tried to scare him away, but he won't go. "

The naturalist smiled and said, "I'll make him leave." So he went into the pen and lifted up the eagle. The eagle was indeed a magnificent bird. He flexed his huge wings, and the naturalist could see some of his latent power. The naturalist said to the eagle, "Stretch forth your wings and fly. You're not a chicken; you're the king of all birds. You can soar over the entire country. Don't be satisfied with this chicken coop." But the eagle plopped down from his arm and went right on pecking for corn just like all the chickens. For days the naturalist kept coming back and putting the eagle on his glove. Still the eagle wouldn't budge.

Finally, exasperated, the naturalist went back to the farmer. "What in the world can I do? That eagle won't budge. He believes he's a chicken."

"Well," the farmer drawled, "if I were you and I had the time, I'd teach him to fly."

The naturalist stared at the farmer for a moment or two. "You know, that's a good idea." So the naturalist put the eagle in a cage and drove his truck to the base of a nearby mountain. He strapped the cage to his back and began to climb the mountain.

He set the cage down on a cliff and opened it, but still the eagle wouldn't budge. He just peered out, blinked, and gazed down at the chickens, far below. The naturalist carefully took the eagle out of the cage and put him on a rock. The eagle looked up at the sky and again his beautiful wings gleamed in the sunlight as they stretched out just a little. For the first time, it seemed that the eagle actually felt different. When he glanced down at the chickens his wings trembled.

The naturalist knew that although the eagle really wanted to fly, he was afraid. So the man reached out and very gently pushed the eagle. It wouldn't budge. He tried again, but still the eagle wouldn't move. Finally, the naturalist sat down, utterly exasperated. He looked at the eagle and at the sky and at the chickens far below. "How can I teach him to fly?" he wondered. Then he happened to glance further up, at the mountaintop, and he knew the answer.

He put the eagle back into the cage and climbed to the very top of the mountain where other eagles roosted. There they built their nests, mated,

raised their offspring, and soared magnificently. The eagle saw all of this
and as soon as the naturalist took him out of the cage, he stretched his gor-
geous wings and eagerly lifted himself off the rock. At first he dropped, but
then he suddenly found, like the other eagles, that he could fly effortlessly.
The eagle never returned to the chicken yard. He had finally discovered who
he was—an eagle. And he loved it.[3]

The dilemma of the eagle is very much the same as ours. We may believe
we are failures when, in truth, we are God's saints by calling, who fail. There
is a big difference. What we believe about ourselves has a tremendous
impact on the way we live our lives. We need to believe about ourselves what
God declares to be true.

What is our identity in Him? For starters, you are much like the eagle,
and God wants you to be free to fly. The story of the eagle beautifully illustrates one of our greatest challenges to living and building our lives in the
present moment. We are often challenged by our own beliefs.

Beliefs profoundly affect the way we act and can end up being a sort of
"self-fulfilling" prophecy. Because the eagle believed he was a chicken, his
perception of reality was distorted. Chickens with chicken beliefs surrounded him and he saw the world through chicken eyes. He thought he
was a chicken, so he acted like a chicken, he lived as a chicken, and in his
heart he was a chicken.

When I thought of myself as a hopeless bulimic, I sank into a pit of
depression and despair. I lived as if that was the core of who I was, feeling
hopeless that things would ever change. When I thought of myself as a
dancer, even though I started very late in life at age twenty-nine, I practiced
diligently and ultimately performed like one. In fact, I *became* a professional
dancer. If you believe you're a chicken, then you'll live like a chicken. If you
believe you're an eagle, then you'll learn to fly.

The second thing this story points out is the power that beliefs have to
trigger our fat machinery. Just as the eagle was limited by his belief that he
was a chicken, you too are limited by all the false beliefs you have about
food, eating, and weight loss. For instance, if you believe that you are a failure and a fat person, you probably eat and act like one. If so, I think we can
safely say that you are not living up to your full potential in Christ. And that
is not God's best for you.

The third insight we gain from this story is that beliefs are rooted in the
past. They have nothing to do with eating from 0 to 5 in present time.

Whatever makes you live like a failure probably happened in the past. Nothing you have done, attempted, or failed to do is beyond the reach and the power of the blood of Jesus.

Failure does not have to have the final word—not where God is concerned. He knows we will fail even before we do, but it is not His will that we fail without benefiting or maturing in some way from the experience. As He applies His grace to our failures, we see an amazing transformation process begin to take shape. We then see that our performance is never the basis of His love for us.

> [We] assume [we] must "try harder" and "do" more to make up for [our] lack of obedience. At this point Grace exclaims, "No. You now live in my realm of freedom, and you have the ever-present strength and help of the Holy Spirit. You must not try harder; you must *strive* less. You must acknowledge your helplessness and total dependence upon the Spirit for your guidance, your area of service, and your ability to love. You are created for good works, but they must flow out of your abiding communion with the Living Vine."[4]

God's grace is more than a pardon; it is a constant, ever-flowing *provision*, a reassuring *presence* and an incredible *power*. Grace washes over and through us, allowing us to experience the redemptive process in all of the ups and downs of our lives.

You are *not* a failure. You are a precious co-heir with Christ, an adopted son or daughter of the Father. God does not want you to remain a chicken. He has given you eagle's wings. Just as the naturalist didn't want to leave the eagle in the chicken coop, your Creator doesn't want you to consider your identity as anything less than it is.

Like an eagle stirs her nest and hovers over its young, that spreads its wings to catch them and carries them on its pinions. The LORD alone led him (Deuteronomy 32:11–12a).

When we are willing to step out of the nest, out of the comfort zones to which we are so attached, failure may seem to loom. However, it is also in those moments that we are also given the opportunity to taste freedom, to experience the Lord God Almighty and His awesome strength as He carries us on His "pinions."

Those who hope in the LORD will renew their strength. They will soar on wings like eagles (Isaiah 40:31a).

The real question is not whether you are going to fail, but rather how you will respond when you do. You may think that there is no hope for you or your situation. As Janice put it, "I was a compulsive overeater and believed I had tried everything possible to get free from this terrible sin, but I always seemed doomed to failure. I felt helpless."

Like many others, Janice was stuck thinking that her failures were bigger than God. This kind of thinking denies the power of the one who rescued us from the greatest of failures, and it denies Paul's declaration, *If God is for us, who can be against us?* (Romans 8:31). We have a Redeemer who loves us, who will forgive us and use our failures to shape and mold us into His likeness. Who else *gives life to the dead and calls things that are not as though they were?* (Romans 4:17b)

Let's take a few moments and examine this a bit more closely.

Take Action

We spoke earlier of different kinds of failure:

+ Failure as a result of leaving God out of the equation.

+ Failure to trust that God is able to do all things.

+ Failure as a result of not being gifted and called by God to a particular endeavor.

In the space below describe one failure that you have experienced and identify which type of failure it is. Then record how God has used that failure to draw you closer to Him, or how He has used it for any other good purpose in your life.

Example:

Perceived Failure: Sarah wrote, "I lost one hundred pounds with a popular weight-loss approach and compulsive exercise but gained back sixty pounds of it."

Failure Type: Sarah wrote, "This failure was a result of the sins of gluttony and denial."

How Used by God: Sarah wrote, "He used that failure to lead me to Thin Within, where I began to develop an intimate relationship with the Lord. As I learned that I could turn to Him for healing of some deeper issues that sent me to food, I released my extra weight, and also quit smoking. What a blessing."

Now apply this to your life.

Perceived Failure: _____

_____

_____

Failure Type: _____

_____

_____

How Used by God: _____

_____

_____

+ Are there things currently happening in your life that you see as failures? If so, offer them to God and ask for His will to be done. Record your thoughts or a prayer request.

_____

_____

_____

Will you choose to receive and thrive on God's love? It bears repeating that we have a God of second, third, fourth, indeed umpteen chances. Rather than see you sink into despair, He longs to have you sink into His loving arms. He will take away any sin, any failure, any mistake and make you clean, so that you can continue on the path of His provision to live a more holy life.

Today, if you find yourself in a situation in which you struggle with success or failure, take a moment to breathe a prayer and ask God:

+ Am I struggling because I have left You out of the equation?
+ Am I struggling because I am not believing that You are able to do all things?
+ Am I struggling as a result of not being called by You for what I'm trying to accomplish?
+ Am I struggling because of willful rebellion?

We can choose to receive God's love, grace, and forgiveness at any moment. While the consequences of our failures may still be evident, we

can allow these experiences to make us more like Christ. Let's choose to live
in the present moment, discovering that God's mercies are new every morning (Lamentations 3:22–23, NRSV).

Your Success Story
Record any new insights you had while reading today.

_____

_____

_____

Verses to Ponder
*Therefore, since we are surrounded by such a great cloud of witnesses, let us
throw off everything that hinders and the sin that so easily entangles, and let
us run with perseverance the race marked out for us. Let us fix our eyes on
Jesus, the author and perfecter of our faith, who for the joy set before him
endured the cross, scorning its shame, and sat down at the right hand of the
throne of God. Consider him who endured such opposition from sinful men, so
that you will not grow weary and lose heart* (Hebrews 12:1–3).

*Therefore, since through God's mercy we have this ministry, we do not lose
heart* (2 Corinthians 4:1).

*We do not want you to be uninformed, brothers, about the hardships we suf-
fered in the province of Asia. We were under great pressure, far beyond our
ability to endure, so that we despaired even of life. Indeed, in our hearts we felt
the sentence of death. But this happened that we might not rely on ourselves
but on God, who raises the dead. He has delivered us from such a deadly peril,
and he will deliver us. On him we have set our hope that he will continue to
deliver us* (2 Corinthians 1:8–10).

Prayer
*Dear Lord, I pray that by the power of Your Holy Spirit, I will allow You
to pick up the pieces when I fail. So often I beat myself up, thinking that
I have failed You and pushed You too far. Forgive me, Lord, for doubt-
ing Your boundless love. I pray that I might learn from my mistakes and
live in present time to honor, obey, and exalt You. In the name of Jesus,
Amen.*

Medical Moment

Even our body knows how to live in present time. Many people are concerned about how often they should eat. One of the most amazing aspects of the body is how it processes its fuel when we are overweight. It actually calls for a small amount of food through the natural hunger and fullness signals. Simultaneously it will use energy that we have stored in the liver and in fat. As we cooperate with our body by eating between 0 and 5, the body will function efficiently while achieving the goal of becoming its God-given size. Overeating and its consequences shorten one's life. When we eat according to these God-given signals, our body functions much more efficiently and will last longer.

—ARTHUR HALLIDAY, M.D.

Success Tools

+ Continue to use the Fat Machinery Log.
+ Fill in the Thin Within Food Log.
+ Mark the Thin Within Observations and Corrections Chart for today.
+ Use the Thin Within Keys to Conscious Eating when you choose to eat or drink today.

Fat Machinery Log

Below, record any of your personal fat machinery ("I paid for it so I should eat all of it"), from others ("You have to clean your plate"), and from the media ("Feed the Need"). As you observe and correct your fat machinery you will be amazed at the changes that will occur in your eating patterns.

Fat Machinery in Me	Fat Machinery from Others	Fat Machinery from Media

Thin Within Food Log

Hunger # before Eating	Time	Items/Amount	Hunger # after Eating

Thin Within Observations and Corrections Chart—Day 10

Observations	Day 10
1. I ate when my body was hungry.	
2. I ate in a calm environment by reducing distractions.	
3. I ate when I was sitting.	
4. I ate when my body and mind were relaxed.	
5. I ate and drank the things my body enjoyed.	
6. I paid attention to my food while eating.	
7. I ate slowly, savoring each bite.	
8. I stopped before my body was full.	

Thin Within Wisdom

God can accomplish much through a "failure" given to Him for His glory!

NOTES

1. Arthur and Judy Halliday, *Thin Again* (Grand Rapids, Michigan: Fleming H. Revell, 1994), 65.
2. Denis Waitley, npa.
3. Original story by Jerry Frankhauser.
4. Cynthia Heald, *Becoming a Woman of Grace* (Nashville: Thomas Nelson Publishers, 1998), 79.

Part II
Enjoying the Development of Discernment

❧

Removal of the Rubble

Humble yourselves, therefore, under God's mighty hand,
that he may lift you up in due time.
Cast all your anxiety on him because he cares for you.
Be self-controlled and alert.
Your enemy the devil prowls around like a roaring lion
looking for someone to devour.
Resist him, standing firm in the faith.
—1 Peter 5:6–9a

The eagle we considered yesterday finally experienced the joy of his true identity. Once he had tasted "eagledom" do you suppose he would ever again return to the chicken coop? Not unless he wanted to enjoy a chicken dinner! Once we understand who we are in Christ, we won't have any reason to look back. In His grace, God has given us a lofty position. He delights in redeeming us. He takes us from the pit in which we dwell apart from Him and lifts us up in Christ. He does all these things for our sake and for the sake of His glory.

When I consider your heavens, the work of your fingers, the moon and the stars, which you have set in place, what is man that you are mindful of him, the son of man that you care for him? You made him a little lower than the heavenly beings and crowned him with glory and honor (Psalm 8:3–5).

As we trust God and give ourselves fully to Him, He demonstrates time and again how trustworthy He is. And as we humble ourselves before the Lord, in His time He lifts us up.

By now we hope you have begun to rest in the fact that your challenges with food, eating, and weight are not hopeless. You have a hope and a future that our God has planned specifically for you. Your old identity is gone, and you have a new identity in Christ (2 Corinthians 5:17). With these truths in mind, let's apply them specifically to your personal Thin Within process. Consider again some of the reasons that you turn to food when you are not at a 0.

1. It's time to eat
2. I'm bored
3. I'm lonely
4. Social pressure
5. Quick energy
6. It's free
7. Etc., etc., etc.

Add to this list any of your own reasons that have not already been identified.

Now let's peel away the superficial layers and focus on the very core of the matter. Since 1975 we have worked with thousands of people at Thin Within. We have learned that a very basic yet powerful belief is in operation for most men and women who struggle with food issues, and here it is:

This is my body, and I can do with it as I please.

You may be saying to yourself, "Well, yes, it is my body." Or, you may be thinking, "I think that way sometimes, but so what?" We have discovered that when struggles with food arise, this belief is always in operation to some degree, although more for some than for others. The extent to which you believe that your body is your own determines whether the reasons for eating listed above (or others like them) cause you to eat when you are not hungry. Let's examine this belief more closely. If we look carefully, we see that it is a big lie.

+ It is a lie that the *Enemy* wants us to believe. Satan is the father of all lies. He prowls around like a roaring lion so that He can devour us. He is, however, defeated as we refuse to believe his lies.

+ It is a lie that the *world* wants us to believe, if for no other reason than to sell us products. It motivates us to seek solutions for our bodies, no matter where we have to go, no matter the extremes we have to endure, no matter how much it costs.

+ It is a lie that *we* want to believe. If we believe it, we don't have to surrender ourselves to God. We don't have to die to the desire to do our will. It is much easier to believe a lie than to give ourselves fully unto the Lord. We struggle with surrender, even in light of all He has given to us.

Perhaps you can relate to Michaela, a Thin Within participant. She complained to a friend about the behavior of her son and his temper tantrums. Her friend replied, "Of course your son has temper tantrums. He sees you having them all the time." When asked to explain, her friend said honestly, "Just think about what you do when you want a double decadent chocolate milkshake. You insist 'I want what I want when I want it' and you head immediately off to the drive-thru."

Michaela's friend was right. We often have temper tantrums about our bodies and our food. "I want what I want when I want it!" Acting very much like spoiled children, we declare in word or deed, "*My* will not Thy will." This is catering to the lie that "my body is my own."

Do you want to restore your temple on a faulty foundation of lies? Or do you want to build on a solid foundation of the truth of God's word? We know that your seeking heart will choose the latter, so let's see how this powerful belief lines up with the word of God.

Do you not know that your body is a temple of the Holy Spirit who is in you, whom you have from God, and that you are not your own? For you have been bought with a price: therefore glorify God in your body (1 Corinthians 6:19–20, NASB).

Consider first the phrase, "Do you not know." God recognizes that we may know this truth in our heads but not in our hearts. As we begin to take captive all of our thoughts that are contrary to Christ's and replace them with the truth of God's Word, we will want to give Him our bodies and our lives. This is a process which at first may not be easy. However, each time we surrender our will and move forward in faith, we will experience God's blessings. Remind yourself that the desire of your flesh is to reserve your body for your own use. God has your ultimate best in mind. Not only are you a temple, a sanctuary in which God has chosen to dwell, but you are set apart by Him and for Him. You are His! He purchased you and therefore you belong to Him—heart, mind, soul, *and* body. This is a *transforming* truth.

However, this truth requires that we submit our will to Him. If we refuse to come to the Lord willingly, it is possible that He will provide the means necessary to cause us to "*be still and* know *that* [He is] God" (Psalm 46:10 emphasis added). It may seem like a "breaking" of our will, but it is always for the purposes set by God in eternity past, something grand and glorious.

Charles Stanley describes it this way: "When my will is eventually saddle-busted completely, then I belong heart, soul, mind, body, spirit, and everything to him. When that happens, my life is totally and completely *His* responsibility. I am His to do with as He pleases. And that, my friend, is when the excitement in life truly begins."[1]

As we surrender ourselves to Him we experience the joy and abundance of a life lived on the edge of adventure. We won't know what comes next, but His provision supplies and equips us for everything to which He calls us. He empowers us to run the race with endurance. We can live in peace, knowing that our lives belong to God, that we are His responsibility. This is true freedom.

God never intends to leave us wounded after He chastens us. Nor does he specifically set out to break our will. He does, however, in all His mercy, allow a measure of suffering so that we will turn to Him and live for His purposes.

In one of his great devotional books, Ken Gire quotes Haddon Robinson, sharing a story about how a shepherd will break the leg of a perpetually wandering sheep. He does this for the purposes of teaching the sheep to stay close by and stop wandering. Mr. Robinson's story concludes, "Many feel that it is an act of cruelty for a shepherd to break the leg of a poor, defenseless sheep. It seems hard-hearted, almost vicious, until you understand the shepherd's heart. Then you realize that what seems to be cruelty is really kindness. The shepherd knows that the sheep must remain close to him if he is to be protected from danger. So he breaks its leg, not to hurt it, but to restore it."[2]

God's word makes it clear that our bodies are not our own and at times drastic measures drive this point home. Nancy, a Thin Within participant, reports that God finally got her attention when she really did break her leg and dislocate her ankle. She realized in a new way that she wasn't as much in control of her life as she had previously believed. She sensed, too, that God wanted her attention so He could point out that she had been turning to food rather than to Him for comfort. As she lay in bed, unable to move without using crutches or a wheelchair, Nancy realized that it was now a lot more trouble to run to the refrigerator. As she turned to the Lord, she released weight effortlessly, even though she was immobile. God met her in that place. The breaking, while painful, was worthwhile.

"This is my body and I can do with it as I please" is a lie that is now exposed by the light of God's Word. Has this lie been pervasive in your life? Once you see the truth, the reasons you eat when you're not hungry may not suddenly disappear, but they will eventually lose their allure.

Take Action

+ In the chart below indicate which of the lies you have believed. Then
using the Bible verse that is listed in the "God's Truth" column, restate
the truth about that lie. An example has been done for you.

The Lie	I Have Believed This Lie	I Have Not Believed This Lie	God's Truth
Example: I can eat as much as want whenever I want it.	X		My body is not my own. I was bought with a price. I am to honor God with my body. (1 Corinthians 6:19–20)
Your turn: I can eat as much as I want whenever I want it.			(Ephesians 5:3; Proverbs 23:20–21)
God doesn't care about my body size or condition.			(Isaiah 40:27)
Eating when I am not hungry isn't important to God.			(James 5:5)
Eating more than my body needs doesn't result in health or emotional problems.			(Proverbs 23:1–3)
The joy I get from eating is worth any suffering that happens as a result.			(Philippians 4:4)
I will worry about getting control of my eating when things aren't so crazy or hectic.			(James 4:13–15)
There is no way anyone can lose weight without cutting out all fat in their foods and working out vigorously at least six times a week.			(1 Corinthians 6:12)

Isn't it amazing how lies can subtly invade our thoughts and become
part of our lives? Our Enemy accuses us night and day before the throne of

God. Please don't allow him to berate, belittle, or defeat you because of the lies you have believed. His intention has been to deceive you and He is a master at it. However, *greater is he that is in you, than he that is in the world* (1 John 4:4, KJV).

Our Lord has purchased your pardon.

Our Lord has purchased your provision.

Our Lord's presence is always at your side.

Our Lord's power is available to you in any moment.

All of this can provide you with the ability to discern truth from error. You may only now be beginning your training in this process, but the Holy Spirit is on the job. If you are a willing student, He will tutor you and you will learn from Him. You have been given everything you need for life and godliness by His very great and precious promises (2 Peter 1:3). He will equip you for the battle. He will go before you, beside you, and behind you. He will never forsake you.

Bible teacher and author, Kay Arthur, says, "Don't struggle in self-effort to be better. Don't determine that you are going to 'try harder.' Acknowledge your need of His all-sufficient grace and go forward, surrendering and trusting in the power of God's transforming grace. 'As you therefore have received Christ Jesus the Lord, so walk in Him' (Colossians 2:6). You were saved by faith; therefore, you are to walk in faith. It may be one step at a time, but walk. You can say, 'I can't,' as long as in the next breath you say, 'But, God, You can.'"[3]

As we continue down this road in the strength He alone can provide, let us walk in truth, tearing down lies that stand as roadblocks before us.

Your Success Story

Record any insights you had while reading today.

_____

_____

_____

Verses to Ponder

O God, you are my God, earnestly I seek you; my soul thirsts for you, my body longs for you, in a dry and weary land where there is no water (Psalm 63:1).

Therefore I tell you, do not worry about your life, what you will eat or drink; or about your body, what you will wear. Is not life more important than food, and the body more important than clothes? (Matthew 6:25)

Do not offer the parts of your body to sin, as instruments of wickedness, but rather offer yourselves to God, as those who have been brought from death to life; and offer the parts of your body to him as instruments of righteousness (Romans 6:13).

So whether you eat or drink or whatever you do, do it all for the glory of God (1 Corinthians 10:31).

Prayer

Dear Lord, I confess that I have acted as if my body belongs to me. I have insisted on eating what I've wanted when I wanted it. Truthfully, Lord, I don't like where I am. I am ready to release my grip on my body and food to You. Please break me where I am proud and strengthen me where I am weak so I can surrender fully to You and to the power of Your transforming grace. I pray that You will cleanse my heart and heal me from within. In Jesus' name, I pray, Amen.

Medical Moment

Living as if we have the right to do with our bodies as we please isn't a wise decision where our physical or spiritual health are concerned. People who disregard the body's God-given signals of hunger and fullness, eating beyond what the body requires, end up with excess weight and are much more likely to suffer from physical and emotional problems. The National Institute of Diabetes and Digestive and Kidney Diseases estimates that in the United States almost seventy percent of heart disease cases are likely linked to excess body fat. Overweight individuals are more likely to develop high blood pressure, breast and colon cancer, and Type 2 diabetes. Additionally, overweight people face a culture with rigid stereotypes that can affect relationships, employment, and educational opportunities. Although this may not be justified, it is often the case. If you have experienced any of these health or emotional problems, perhaps you have additional reasons for considering offering your body to the One who created it for His will and control. In this place of absolute surrender, there is an opportunity for wholeness and improved health.

—Arthur Halliday, M.D.

Success Tools

- ✦ Use the Thin Within Food Log.
- ✦ Continue to use the Fat Machinery Log.
- ✦ Mark the Thin Within Observations and Corrections Chart for today.
- ✦ Use the Thin Within Keys to Conscious Eating every time you choose to eat or drink today.

Thin Within Food Log

Hunger # before Eating	Time	Items/Amount	Hunger # after Eating

Fat Machinery Log

Below, record any of your personal fat machinery ("I paid for it so I should eat all of it"), from others ("You have to clean your plate"), and from the media ("Feed the Need"). As you observe and correct your fat machinery you will be amazed at the changes that will occur in your eating patterns.

Fat Machinery in Me	Fat Machinery from Others	Fat Machinery from Media

Thin Within Observations and Corrections Chart—Day 11

Observations	Day 11
1. I ate when my body was hungry.	
2. I ate in a calm environment by reducing distractions.	
3. I ate when I was sitting.	
4. I ate when my body and mind were relaxed.	
5. I ate and drank the things my body enjoyed.	
6. I paid attention to my food while eating.	
7. I ate slowly, savoring each bite.	
8. I stopped before my body was full.	

Thin Within Wisdom

Ask the Lord to reveal where your "fat machinery" is in operation. He is faithful and He will do it!

NOTES

1. Charles Stanley, *The Blessings of Brokenness* (Grand Rapids, Michigan: Zondervan Publishing House, 1997), 64.
2. © 1988 Cook Communications Ministries. *Reflections on the Word* by Ken Gire. Reprinted with permission. May not be further reproduced. All rights reserved.
3. Kay Arthur, *Lord, I Need Grace to Make It* (Sisters, Oregon: Multnomah Books, 1989), 113.

⤜⤝

Furnishing the Halls of the Mind

*Those who carried materials did their work with
one hand and held a weapon in the other,
and each of the builders wore his sword at his side as he worked.*
—Nehemiah 4:17b–18a

God has done great works through His people throughout history. After Jerusalem was destroyed by enemies, He rebuilt His holy city through the Israelites. Nehemiah and the Jewish workers rebuilt the wall around Jerusalem following the return of the exiles from Babylon. Like the workers in Nehemiah's day, we have hammers in our right hands and swords strapped to our sides. We want to protect the work God is doing in our rebuilding process.

If you don't know by now, you will soon find out that there are potential detractors in the rebuilding process, and you need to be vigilant and refuse to let the Enemy into the camp. Follow the example of the returned exiles by strapping on the "sword of the Spirit" (Ephesians 6:17). God's Word will continue to direct you as He powerfully places each and every building block in the restoration of your body, His temple.

Do not conform any longer to the pattern of this world, but be transformed by the renewing of your mind. Then you will be able to test and approve what God's will is—his good, pleasing and perfect will (Romans 12:2).

Our minds are being renewed according to the truth of God's Word. Yesterday we identified some lies that have kept you from experiencing God's best. The cornerstone of overcoming lies with truth is to realize that God doesn't see us as we see ourselves. He sees us in Him, as more than conquerors.

Once our lives were based on what we accepted as truth, but now we have found the truth in His Word. The Enemy, however, is always there to make us feel uncertain about the ground on which we stand. Vulnerable as we are, we need to rally together and stand faithful to the call of God. Today we will identify and learn how to deal with the "hecklers" that will present detours or roadblocks meant to deter us from the work God is doing.

As the returned exiles began to rebuild the wall around Jerusalem, they found themselves faced with those who wanted to intimidate or distract them. This is why the builders worked with tools in one hand and a weapon in the other. Under Nehemiah's guidance, they remained vigilant against such possibilities. We must do the same.

Our first taunting cynic is Larry the Legalist. Larry claims that we have no business building with such freedom. Can you hear him? "You aren't counting calories, or weighing and measuring your food," he protests. "What kind of food log is *that*?"

Perhaps in the past you might have found yourself in the camp with the legalists, but now you have rid yourself of such entanglements. Legalists will even try to persuade you that the Thin Within approach is no way to release excess weight. They may insist instead on such things as logging your exercise minutes and heart rate every day, then calculating a direct comparison of weight versus calories ingested or other such formulaic ways of arriving at your weight goal.

The above approach, as you know by now, will derail your efforts to walk on the path of God's provision. Larry the Legalist is caught on the path of his own performance. Many of us have been there and know that on that path we may experience temporary "success." But unfortunately the success never lasts. To make matters worse, it is on that path of our performance that the "club of condemnation" appears at every turn. This is not what Christ died to give us. He died to give us freedom.

On the path of our performance we feel like we're in control. We humans like to feel that way. But as we saw yesterday, control does not belong to us. The Lord purchased us to be His and with our new identity in Christ, legalism and fixed formulas are incompatible with our freedom. Our tendency is to cling to familiar rules to follow. We like the familiarity of the legalistic approach and feel drawn toward the food plans Larry recommends. This is illustrated for you in figure 12-1.

Larry likes control, so counting calories and fat grams gives him a sense that he is in charge. Under the confines of the law, he knows the rules, what is expected of him, and the standards for his performance. He wants to take us with him, but this is the detour that leads off God's path and back to the path of our performance. Do we really want to go there? Of course not. Why? Because Larry's way does not work!

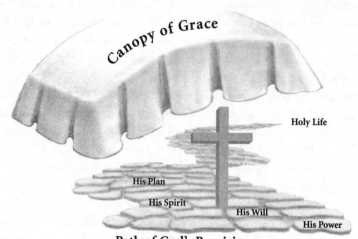

Path of God's Provision
Two Steps Forward and One Back • Leading Toward the Holy Life • Confidence in God

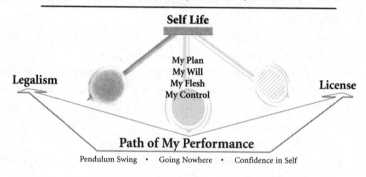

Path of My Performance
Pendulum Swing • Going Nowhere • Confidence in Self

figure 12–1

"The disciple living by grace rather than law has undergone a decisive conversion—*a turning from mistrust to trust.* The foremost characteristic of living by grace is trust in the redeeming work of Jesus Christ,"[1] says Brennan Manning.

If Larry's legalistic approach doesn't work, Maureen the Manipulator may come along with her backdoor approach. "OK," she says, "have your 0 to 5 eating. But shouldn't you at least eat diet foods when you're hungry? Think of the results you'll get if you combine Thin Within with all low-fat foods." As if to drive home her point, Maureen says, "That would be doing it 'God's way' and the way that makes sense. You can't fail."

What is our response to Maureen and Larry?

It is for freedom that Christ has set us free. Stand firm, then, and do not let yourselves be burdened again by a yoke of slavery (Galatians 5:1).

Larry the Legalist and Maureen the Manipulator are perfectly aware of the fact that Americans love diets and diet foods; they love commandments and laws about their eating. Yet obesity continues to be a raging epidemic. We have the most food of any country in the world and the most diets to keep us from eating it.

I found that the very commandment that was intended to bring life actually brought death (Romans 7:10).

The very commandments about food that are intended to bring life have actually brought death. The more low-fat foods we eat, the more full-fat foods we want. Often eating half the calories of the original product just means we end up eating twice as much and then some. Food formulas seem so great. If we perform just right, we "lose" the weight, but once we stop the performance, we almost always "find" the weight again. We are either puffed up because of how well we perform (weight lost) or depressed because of how poorly we perform (weight found), and neither state offers permanent results.

Food formulas point the finger at the food but not at the heart. And that leads us to another heckler. Abigail the Achiever joined us on Day One of our journey. She has applied the keys to conscious eating and has found herself releasing weight faster than she can run out to buy smaller pants to fit her new body. She loves the freedom of Thin Within and enjoys having people notice how well she is doing. Abigail has begun to glow in the glory of her "achievement." Abigail has begun to "strut her stuff," proudly displaying her thinner body. She is "in control" and loves it.

Do you notice how Abigail went from freedom to a form of legalism? She went from God-control to flesh-control. How did this switch occur? In a word, the answer is pride. Abigail is beginning to take a detour off of the path of God's provision and onto the path of her performance. She received her freedom by being in Christ, yet now she is beginning to take all the credit. What began in the Spirit, she is now trying to complete in the flesh, giving glory to herself.

Abigail has begun to think that she has "arrived." She considers herself a notch above others spiritually because she has proven to herself, to God, and to the world that she can release weight by her self-effort alone. She appears to have forgotten that it is the Lord who purchased her freedom. It is the Lord who has exposed the lie of her former beliefs and it is the Lord who has equipped her to act in accordance with His truth.

Brennan Manning asks "How long will it be before we discover we cannot dazzle God with our accomplishments? When will we acknowledge that we need not and cannot buy God's favor? When will we acknowledge that we don't have it all together and happily accept the gift of grace? When will we grasp the thrilling truth of Paul: 'We acknowledge that what makes a man righteous is not obedience to the Law, but faith in Jesus Christ'" (Galatians 2:16)?[2]

Let us not be distracted by Larry, Maureen, or Abigail. Instead let us remain committed to Christ, allowing Him to conform us more to His will from *within*. We must accept our new identity in Christ. Only then can we fully experience the sacrificial life He has given us.

In her book, *Lord, I Need Grace to Make It*, Kay Arthur says, "The Law was never intended to make a man or woman righteous, whether he or she was a lost person or a saved person. If you and I can remember this truth, it will forever cast us upon His grace. Grace will become the key that will unlock a life of greater peace, trust, confidence, obedience, and intimacy with our heavenly Father and His Son as we walk hand in hand with the Spirit of Grace."[3]

The entire purpose of the law was to prove that we couldn't pull off the business of living without His help. We need God's grace to make it. The law was given so that we would discover that there has to be some other way. And there is another way. Christ is the way.

So the law was put in charge to lead us to Christ that we might be justified by faith. Now that faith has come, we are no longer under the supervision of the law (Galatians 3:24–25).

Once we are in Christ, we are under grace instead of the law. But what does it mean to be "in Christ"? What does that look like in my everyday life?

"In Christ," I am inspired by His Spirit *to will and to work for His good pleasure* (Ephesians 1:9, NASB).

"In Christ," I am equipped for whatever He calls me to do, and I am empowered to *fight the good fight, holding on to faith and a good conscience* (1 Timothy 1:18b–19a).

"In Christ," I eat only when I am truly hungry and I stop before I am full. I am not obsessed by counting calories or fat grams. As I eat, I praise God for His goodness. I am free, no longer a slave to sin (Romans 6:6). I am raised up to live a new life of glorious freedom (Romans 6:4). I praise and glorify Christ, not myself. I love practicing the presence of God, walking in fellowship with Him moment by moment. It is truly the icing on the cake that I am releasing weight as well.

When we die to the law and come under grace, like the chicken-coop eagle being given the freedom to fly, we are set free to live the abundant, holy life. But it is important to note that grace is not a license for indulging our sensual pleasures. Christina said it well: "I call it 'greasy grace' when I abuse one of God's greatest gifts by sliding into a casual, comfortable life knowing that whatever I do will be forgiven." God's word drives this point firmly home:

What shall we say, then? Shall we go on sinning so that grace may increase? By no means! We died to sin; how can we live in it any longer? (Romans 6:1–2)

We don't treat the grace of God with contempt by turning it into a license to do whatever we please. We respond with love and gratitude to the goodness of God and His pardon, provision, presence, and power.

"To teach grace is to teach a full and complete dependence upon God to provide according to His infinite love all that is needed by the one who places trust in Him. The life of such a one must be a God-directed life. And a God-directed life is not one of carelessness and license. There is no indifference to sin in such a life. Only under grace can such a life be lived."[4]

So, then, how are we to live under grace and not under the law when it comes to our eating habits? We are free to choose to have chocolate if we are hungry, but as we progress further along with our restoration project, we will see that grace also means being free not to eat chocolate.

I have learned that grace gives me the freedom to refuse or choose a particular food. It means I am free from chains, free to hear the voice of the Spirit leading and directing me. I don't need to be afraid that "this is the last helping of chocolate Oreo chip ice cream so I better eat it now before someone else gets it." Grace says that I will gladly share because I can buy another quart of the same flavor any time I choose.

In the words of Jeanelle, "At Thin Within I learned about conscious eating and I applied the keys, but the most important gift I received was grace—grace with myself and with others. My stomach knots loosened when I accepted God's grace into my life."

Will you accept God's grace? The path of His provision is a blessed place of freedom, rest, obedience, and peace that leads us to holy living. As Neil

Anderson, author of *Victory Over Darkness*, puts it, "The grace to let go and let God be God flows from trust in His boundless love."[5]

Take Action

+ In the chart below, use an X to identify whether each thought goes along with the law or goes along with grace. (Answers are given at the end of the Day Twelve chapter.)

Thought	Law	Grace
1. I am hungry now, but I ate too much at lunch. I better not eat now.		
2. I am hungry now, but I can choose to wait until my lunch date with Donna to eat.		
3. I just ate a small bowl of cereal. Am I past a 5? Oh shoot, I think I am past a 5. Shucks. I know I am past a 5. I blew it!		
4. I need an abundance of carbohydrates, fats and protein each day, so even though I am not hungry, I better be sure to eat something right now.		
5. That's funny. I just ate a small meal two hours ago. I know I am at a zero. I better not eat, though. I could never lose weight if I did that.		
6. I love being able to eat chocolate again if I choose or leave it if I choose.		
7. If I eat to a 6 I have blown my Thin Within eating program.		

✦ Read the following, which will help you see who you are in Christ. As you read, praise God for all He has done and provided for you in Christ.

Who I Am In Christ

I am God's child for I am born again of the incorruptible
seed of the Word of God which lives and abides forever..... 1 Pet. 1:23

I am forgiven all my sins and washed in the blood .... Eph. 1:7

I am a new creature .... 2 Cor. 5:17

I am a temple of the Holy Spirit .... 1 Cor. 6:19

I am delivered from the power of darkness and
transformed into God's kingdom....................... Col. 1:13

I am redeemed from the curse of the law.................... Gal. 3:13

I am strong in the Lord................................. Eph. 6:10

I am holy and without blame before Him.................... Eph. 1:4

I am accepted in Christ................................. Eph. 1:6

I am blessed.. Deut. 28:1–14

I am a saint .... Rom. 1:7

I am qualified to share in His inheritance................... Col. 1:12

I am the head and not the tail; I am above only
and not beneath .... Deut. 28:13

I am victorious...................................... Rev. 21:7

I am dead to sin .... Rom. 6: 2, 11

I am elect.. Col. 3:12

I am loved with an everlasting love .... Jer. 31:3

I am established to the end .... 1 Cor. 1:8

I am set free .... Jn. 8:31–33

I am circumcised with the circumcision made without hands ... Col. 2:11

I am crucified with Christ.............................. Gal. 2:20

I am alive with Christ................................. Eph. 2:5

I am raised up with Christ and seated in heavenly places .... Col. 2:12

I am His faithful follower.............................. Eph. 5:1

I am the light of the world .... Matt. 5:14

I am the salt of the earth.............................. Matt. 5:13

I am called of God.................................... 2 Tim. 1:9

I am brought near by the blood of Christ .... Eph. 2:13

I am more than a conqueror............................ Rom. 8:37

I am in Christ Jesus by His doing .... 1 Cor. 1:30

I am an ambassador for Christ .... 2 Cor. 5:20
I am beloved of God .... 1 Thess. 1:4
I am the first fruits among His creation .... Jas. 1:18
I am born of God and the evil one does not touch me .... 1 Jn. 5:18
I am a king and a priest unto God .... Rev. 1:6
I am a joint heir with Christ .... Rom. 8:17
I am reconciled to God. .... 2 Cor. 5:18
I am overtaken with blessings .... Deut. 28:2
I am healed by the wounds of Jesus .... 1 Pet. 2:24
I am in the world as He is in heaven .... 1 Jn. 4:17
I am a fellow citizen with the saints
    of the household of God .... Eph. 2:19
I am sealed with the promise of the Holy Spirit .... Eph. 1:13
I am complete in Christ. .... Col. 2:10
I am the apple of my Father's eye .... Ps. 17:8
I am free from condemnation. .... Rom. 8:1
I am the righteousness of God through Jesus Christ. .... 2 Cor. 5:21
I am chosen. .... 1 Thess. 1:4
I am firmly rooted, built up, strengthened in the faith and
    overflowing with thankfulness .... Col. 2:7
I am a disciple of Christ because
    I have love for others .... Jn. 13:34–35
I am built on the foundations of the apostles and prophets,
    with Christ Jesus Himself as the chief cornerstone .... Eph. 2:20
I am a partaker of His divine nature .... 2 Pet. 1:4
I am God's workmanship, created in Christ Jesus
    for good works .... Eph. 2:10
I am being changed into His image .... Phil. 1:6
I am one in Christ! Hallelujah! .... Jn. 17:21–23
I have all my needs met by God according to his
    glorious riches in Christ Jesus .... Phil. 4:19
I have the mind of Christ. .... 1 Cor. 2:16
I have everlasting life .... Jn. 6:47
I have a guaranteed inheritance .... Eph. 1:14
I have abundant life .... Jn. 10:10
I have overcome the world .... 1 Jn. 5:4
I have the peace of God which passes understanding .... Phil. 4:7

I have access to the Father by one Spirit .... Eph. 2:18
I can do all things through Jesus Christ.................... Phil. 4:13
I walk in Christ Jesus...................................... Col. 2:6
I press toward the goal for the prize of the high calling of God .. Phil. 3:14
I live by the law of the Holy Spirit .... Rom. 8:2
I know God's voice.. Jn. 10:14
I show forth His praise .... 1 Pet. 2:9
I always triumph in Christ............................... 2 Cor. 2:14
CHRIST IS IN ME, THE HOPE OF GLORY!................ Col. 1:27[6]

God has made a great exchange—His life for ours. He has attributed a new identity to those who are in Christ. We are not made righteous by the law, but only because He chose us before the foundation of the world. Stand firm today as one who has been made new. God is at work in you, continuing to make you perfect and holy in Him.

Your Success Story

Record new insights while reading today.

_____

_____

_____

Verses to Ponder

For sin shall not be your master, because you are not under law, but under grace (Romans 6:14).

And God is able to make all grace abound to you, so that in all things at all times, having all that you need, you will abound in every good work (2 Corinthians 9:8).

But he said to me, "My grace is sufficient for you, for my power is made perfect in weakness." Therefore I will boast all the more gladly about my weaknesses, so that Christ's power may rest on me (2 Corinthians 12:9).

I do not set aside the grace of God, for if righteousness could be gained through the law, Christ died for nothing! (Galatians 2:21)

Prayer

Lord, I have been at times tempted to return to what is familiar. Please forgive me. Help me to trust more in You and Your grace. Help me never to return to the bondage of food or eating laws. I want to trust You and Your word more completely. I pray that I will lean on You and not on my own understanding as I walk in obedience under the grace You have so freely given. In Jesus' name, Amen.

Medical Moment

Dissemination of medical information has never been more widespread than at the present time through journals, books, health newsletters, magazines, newspapers, and the Internet. What is perhaps not well appreciated is that there is a rapid turnover in medical "facts." Approximately fifty percent of what we believe today will turn out not to be true five years from now. It is therefore important that we avoid clinging to outmoded ideas or accepting as fact something that does not stand up to scientific scrutiny. And while it is always wise to be open to new ideas relating to health and fitness, it is also very wise to be cautious of "far-out" solutions to our problems. Nowhere is this more important than in the "health industry" where many strange and even bizarre "miracle cures" appear weekly. The focus of any weight-management program should be on our internal physical, emotional, and spiritual health, which in turn will be manifested externally in a body that reflects the glory of God.

—ARTHUR HALLIDAY, M.D.

Success Tools
+ Fill in the Thin Within Food Log.
+ Mark the Thin Within Observations and Corrections Chart for today.
+ Use the Thin Within Keys to Conscious Eating today.

Thin Within Wisdom
The path of God's provision is a path of freedom.

Thin Within Food Log

Hunger # before Eating	Time	Items/Amount	Hunger # after Eating

Thin Within Observations and Corrections Chart—Day 12

Observations	Day 12
1. I ate when my body was hungry.	
2. I ate in a calm environment by reducing distractions.	
3. I ate when I was sitting.	
4. I ate when my body and mind were relaxed.	
5. I ate and drank the things my body enjoyed.	
6. I paid attention to my food while eating.	
7. I ate slowly, savoring each bite.	
8. I stopped before my body was full.	

NOTES

1. Brennan Manning, *The Ragamuffin Gospel* (Sisters, Oregon: Multnomah Books, 2000), 74.
2. ibid, 138.
3. Kay Arthur, *Lord, I Need Grace to Make It* © 1989 Kay Arthur.
4. John F. Strombeck, *Grace and Truth* (Grand Rapids, Michigan: Kregel Publications, 1991), 76–77.
5. Neil Anderson, *Victory Over Darkness*, © 2000. Regal Books. Used by permission.
6. Mark TeVogt as quoted in pamphlet, *Who I Am in Christ*, (Cincinnati, Ohio: Christian Information Committee, 2000), 1–3.

Answers to the Law and Grace Exercise:

1. Law
2. Grace
3. Law
4. Law
5. Law
6. Grace
7. Law

Wind Beneath My Wings

You yourselves have seen what I did to Egypt,
and how I carried you on eagles' wings and brought you to myself.
—Exodus 19:4

Once you have tasted the sky,
You will walk the earth with your eyes skyward.
For you have been there,
And there, you will return.
—Leonardo da Vinci

Once we have begun to experience freedom, there really won't be any looking back. The Lord is freeing us from slavery to the past, to the lies we have believed, to our fat machinery, to unconscious eating patterns, and to legalism or the law. He has been removing rubble and laying a foundation—the foundation, of course, is Christ Himself.

Joy begins to fill our hearts as we refuse to take on any identity except the one He purchased for us. Who are you in Him? Your identity is found not in your performance, but only in Him.

Our salvation is signed, sealed, and delivered instantly upon receiving His gift, which was purchased by Jesus on Calvary's cross. But walking in the newness of this life doesn't happen all at once. The intimacy God wants to share with us increases as we release to Him our unmet needs and our expectations of others and ourselves. It occurs by degrees as we surrender our mind, emotions, and will to Him. It occurs in obedience to His will as we look to Him moment by moment for inspiration and accept His equipping and His empowerment. He intends that His grace should infuse every aspect of our lives.

We've learned the hard way that living in the flesh doesn't work. Now that we have accepted our freedom, we must begin to develop discernment and choose whether to serve the flesh or live the Spirit-led life.

For when we were controlled by the sinful nature, the sinful passions aroused by the law were at work in our bodies, so that we bore fruit for death (Romans 7:5).

We now need to practice taking our every thought captive (2 Corinthians 10:5). In the past our runaway thoughts led us to think about and lust for food even when we weren't hungry. Now we will be very attentive to what we are thinking moment by moment because it is clear that our previous eating habits literally bore fruit for death through high blood pressure, diabetes, heart disease, and other similar maladies. Dieting laws or messages from our culture have loudly proclaimed that our worth is determined by our appearance, fueling the very beliefs that result in inappropriate eating. Thankfully we have been released from the laws of the past.

But now, by dying to what once bound us, we have been released from the law so that we serve in the new way of the Spirit, and not in the old way of the written code (Romans 7:6).

Paul says, "We have been released from the law." It is something that has been done. Past tense. We don't need to await the freedom. We have it. We can live in the Spirit now, today, this minute. Why do we at times resist waiting until we reach that 0 or insist on eating beyond 5? Why do we eat when we are not hungry? Let's look at the apostle Paul's rendering of the battle that we face:

I do not understand what I do. For what I want to do I do not do, but what I hate I do (Romans 7:15).

William Well-Meaning identifies with this battle. He wakes up, ready to start his day with his Bible, his *Thin Within* book, and his journal. He prays, studies, reads, and after a wonderful time of fellowship and communion with the Lord, he heads off to work, having promised the Lord that *today* will be different. *Today* he will give his body to God and live for Him. *Today* he will eat 0 to 5, being fully convinced that this will honor the Lord. Then what? William Well-Meaning, before he knows it, finds himself snacking on one thing or another, ultimately realizing that he is walking in the flesh. The very thing he didn't want to do, the very thing he hates is what he finds himself doing.

The apostle Paul loved the Lord very much and was used by Him in a mighty way. Yet he confessed a similar struggle:

I know that nothing good lives in me, that is, in my flesh. For I have the desire to do what is good, but I cannot carry it out. For what I do is not the good I want to do; no, the evil I do not want to do—this I keep on doing (Romans 7:18–19).

Paul reverted from the Spirit back to the flesh or the law. Can you identify with this struggle? Perhaps like William Well-Meaning you have been caught up in a similar cycle, and by three o'clock in the afternoon you end up throwing your hands in the air, disappointed in the demise of your good intentions. If so, be encouraged by Paul's words.

William has, without realizing it, bought the lies of Larry the Legalist. He has begun to revert to the law. But William will discover what Paul clarifies for us—there is no power in the law to change us. William can jump off of the path of my performance and begin afresh on the path of God's provision by applying the tool of observation and correction. We've illustrated this for you in figure 13-1.

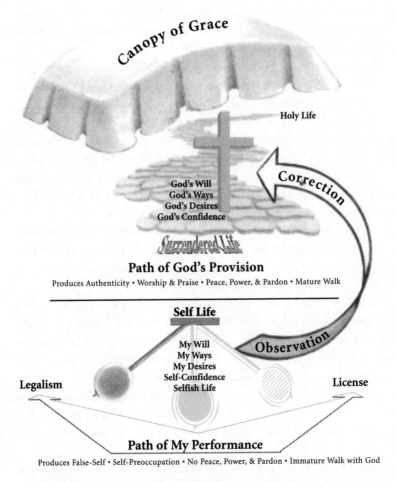

figure 13-1

In Romans 7, Paul applied this principle.

So I find this law at work: When I want to do good, evil is right there with me. For in my inner being I delight in God's law; but I see another law at work in the members of my body, waging war against the law of my mind and making me a prisoner of the law of sin at work within my members. What a wretched man I am! Who will rescue me from this body of death? (Romans 7:21–24)

Paul saw what he was doing and made the proper correction. After reverting to the law, he realized that trying to keep the law through self-effort was futile because his flesh was weak. His hope lay elsewhere, in Christ. He concluded that he was stuck with a body bent on death. The only power to live effectively in newness of life is found in surrendering to the Spirit of God. So, what did Paul say next?

Thanks be to God—through Jesus Christ our Lord! (Romans 7:25)

There is good reason for gratitude once the correction is made and we focus our eyes on Him. Paul realized that his proper identity was in Christ. He recognized that without the Spirit all he could count on was failure. But he didn't accept the identity of a "failure." He recognized that he was no longer a slave to sin, but was now a slave to God, even if his body sometimes behaved otherwise. He thanked God that the truth lies in Christ through whom Paul was set free. Like him, once we are in Christ we have the freedom to become instruments of righteousness (Romans 6:13).

Yes, there is a battle. But the law of the Spirit of life has set us free from reverting constantly back to the law of sin and death. We can resist our tendency to gravitate toward the law, standing firm on our true identity as we continue to observe and correct. Let's keep at it.

We will face battles and challenges, but anything this valuable is worth the fight. Call on Him and He will answer. His Spirit will inspire you, enable you, and empower you to fight in the strength He provides. With an act of your will and a sincere heart, you can call out for help in any moment, in any temptation. He has promised to come to your aid.

No temptation has seized you except what is common to man. And God is faithful; he will not let you be tempted beyond what you can bear. But when you are tempted, he will also provide a way out so that you can stand up under it (1 Corinthians 10:13).

God will not fail to keep His promise to provide you with a way out of temptation. He will continue to help you no matter how many times you cry out, "Lord, I am sorry. I did it again." No matter how often you find yourself on your face before Him, He will always, always, always offer His hand, lift you up, embrace you, brush away your tears, cleanse you and give you a clean robe of righteousness. He is the wind beneath your wings which lift you up. Will you soar with Him?

Take Action

Think of a naturally thin person, someone who is not governed by rules or laws regarding food and eating. People like this don't work at being their natural size. They haven't reached that size by following laws or formulas. Their relationship to food and eating flows freely. They provide a picture of freedom and hope that God has for you.

A naturally thin person is a living example of the keys to conscious eating in action; her success isn't due to low-fat eating, the counting of calories, or excessive exercise. The credit would be misplaced if she attributed to the law (dieting and exercise rules) something she has experienced naturally.

God has designed you with all that you need to be a naturally thin person. Free from food rules your confidence needn't come from your own efforts but from the life of Christ within you.

Observing the Behavior of Thin People Exercise

Consider a naturally thin person that you know, someone who is thin from within. Such a person does not struggle with food, eating, or the body. They do have other struggles, however, because the Bible reassures us that every person experiences trials and temptations.

Naturally thin people seem instinctively to eat between 0 and 5. They don't eat only diet foods, and they eat anything they want when they are hungry. Observe the behavior of the naturally thin person you know and record your observations of how that thin person relates to food, eating, and his or her body.

The Behavior of My Naturally Thin Friend

_____

_____

_____

_____

A Thin Within participant, Teri, tells of her sister's eating habits: "She always eats small amounts, making a huge deal out of each bite, as she moves the food around in her mouth. I never could understand it before. Also, she is quite happy taking a single bite of someone else's chocolate mousse pie instead of ordering her own. She eats strange things at odd hours. She always leaves food on her plate. It seems as if she never eats much of anything at a sitting, but you can tell she really enjoys whatever she eats. When I asked her about when she eats she said, 'When I'm hungry.' She's been living and using the Keys to Conscious Eating all her life."

Take a minute to evaluate your own behavior over the past twelve days. Look at all those places on your Observations and Corrections Charts that have your special marks. Do you see that you have been applying yourself to some degree to eating like Teri's sister? Celebrate all the times you have practiced Spirit-filled eating. Give thanks to God for all those times you relied on the Spirit and took a stand against your flesh. Each mark on each chart represents a "win" for the glory of God.

The fact that you have chosen to fight indicates that you are making choices according to the leading of the Holy Spirit. Observe and correct the things that stand in the way of reaching your godly goals. Surrender yourself to the Lord and let Him take control once again. If you find you are flesh-controlled, stop and ask God to fill all your empty places with Himself. You can leave your fat machinery behind, soaring higher on the wind beneath your wings.

Your Success Story

Did you have any new insights while you were reading today? Please record them below.

_____

_____

_____

Verses to Ponder

I led them with cords of human kindness, with ties of love; I lifted the yoke from their neck and bent down to feed them (Hosea 11:4).

The LORD appeared to us in the past, saying: "I have loved you with an everlasting love; I have drawn you with loving-kindness" (Jeremiah 31:3).

Prayer

Thank You, Lord, that I can live in the Spirit by Your grace alone, which is extended freely to me through the blood of Jesus. Thank You for being at work in me and that I am making progress with You. Help me to lean on You and not to give in to my fleshly desires. Help me to call out to You in my moments of temptation and to have the faith that You will lead me in the ways that I should go. In Jesus' name I pray, Amen.

Medical Moment

Concerns with the pressures of our society and the overemphasis on appearance by the media have caused an increase in three eating disorders in this country during the past thirty years. Anorexia is defined as weighing fifteen percent or more below one's ideal body weight; bulimia is characterized by binge eating followed by self-induced vomiting and/or excessive use of laxatives or diuretics; and there is binge eating without purging. These disorders, which are now being seen in children even under the age of ten, have potentially serious physical, spiritual, and psychological consequences. They require early recognition and multidisciplinary treatment that focuses on many facets of the person's life, personality, and relationships. An important component of the healing process is for the person to achieve a godly perspective of his or her body, food and eating, and a clear understanding of issues regarding self-identity. When eating disorders are addressed on an emotional, physical, and spiritual basis, we observe profound results for long-term recovery.

—ARTHUR HALLIDAY, M.D.

Success Tools

- ✦ Fill in the Thin Within Food Log.
- ✦ Mark the Thin Within Observations and Corrections Chart.
- ✦ Use the Thin Within Keys to Conscious Eating when you choose to eat or drink today.

Thin Within Wisdom

The law of the Spirit of life sets us free from giving in to the lusts of our flesh. We can then become the size that He intends us to be!

Thin Within Food Log

Hunger # before Eating	Time	Items/Amount	Hunger # after Eating

Thin Within Observations and Corrections Chart—Day 13

Observations	Day 13
1. I ate when my body was hungry.	
2. I ate in a calm environment by reducing distractions.	
3. I ate when I was sitting.	
4. I ate when my body and mind were relaxed.	
5. I ate and drank the things my body enjoyed.	
6. I paid attention to my food while eating.	
7. I ate slowly, savoring each bite.	
8. I stopped before my body was full.	

Choosing to Build on Truth

He has made perfect forever those who are being made holy.
—Hebrews 10:14b

Much has transpired on this road to freedom, and many lessons are still being learned as we drink deeply from God's river of grace. We pray that your thirsty soul is refreshed and that you are strengthened for continuing on the scenic path that leads to the holy life in Christ.

Recall our parable about the eagle in the chicken coop. Who has God created you to be? Do you ever find yourself acting like a chicken, even though *you* are, in truth, an eagle? However, unless you choose to believe that you *are* an eagle, you won't spread your wings and soar as God intended.

God enables us to see that in fact we are eagles, made and redeemed in Christ. He inspires us to believe and He equips us with the wings required for flight.

Yet there are important aspects of our identity as an eagle in which we participate. First, we must *believe* that we are meant to fly. Second, we must *act* on that belief, trusting that, as we spread our wings, the wind will, in fact, sustain us. Our beliefs lay the foundation for our actions as seen in figure 14-1.

If God had not intended the eagle to fly, stepping off the cliff with or without wings spread would have proven disastrous!

Let us look closely at who we are in Christ so that our beliefs are based solidly upon the truth.

At the Cross our old self was buried with Christ, so that just as Christ was raised from the dead, we too, might live a new life (Romans 6:4). Our body of sin was done away with, rendered powerless, so that we are no longer slaves of sin. Our identity was fundamentally changed by what Christ accomplished on the cross (Romans 6:6).

If we believe these truths, it will profoundly affect our subsequent behaviors. Romans 6:11 exhorts us to consider ourselves dead to sin, but alive to God. How does a dead person respond to an "opportunity" to sin? Well, he doesn't! Exactly! That is how we can now respond to temptation in our lives, knowing that God has provided a way out (1 Corinthians 10:13).

What I believe about myself affects how I act. The old me died in Christ. The new me was given birth when Jesus rose from the grave. *Therefore, if anyone is in Christ, he is a new creation; the old has gone, the new has come!* (2 Corinthians 5:17).

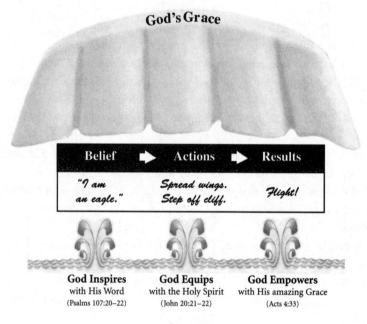

figure 14–1

Because of this fundamental change in who I am, I can respond to Paul's request, *Do not offer the parts of your body to sin, as instruments of wickedness, but rather offer yourselves to God, as those who have been brought from death to life; and offer the parts of your body to him as instruments of righteousness* (Romans 6:13).

I really *can* choose in this minute to put to death the deeds of the flesh and say no to another piece of pecan pie. I am no longer compelled to sin! I am free to *offer* my body to God for righteousness.

We have a new master. Sin no longer rules us because we are now under grace (Romans 6:14). We have been set free from the bondage to sin and have become slaves to God. This leads to holiness and eternal life (Romans 6:22). Our Lord imparts newness of life to us through the Spirit of Christ, which gives us the power to make holy choices. He inspires us to believe Him; He equips us to act.

We can confidently choose to lift our wings upon this truth, letting the winds of grace catch us, or we can hold our feathers in tight to our bodies, refusing to believe that we are, in fact, eagles, destined for the sky.

Fly with us, dear reader! Build your life on the truth that God has declared about you. You are His chosen one. You are holy in Him. This is who you are. You are not a chicken made for scratching in the chicken coop. You are an eagle, born to rule the sky. Believe in God's power, God's grace, and God's will for you and stretch forth your wings. Fly!

Colossians 3:12 states, *You are God's chosen people, holy and dearly loved.* In this verse and in many others in the New Testament, you are identified as *holy and dearly loved.* You are holy. This is a fact based on God's provision, purpose, plan, and pardon. He chose you to be holy and blameless in His sight before the foundation of the world (Ephesians 1:4).

Not only that, but you are being made holy day by day as you give the right of way to the Holy Spirit within (Hebrews 10:14).

"But," you may object, "I have binged three times in the last six days. How can I possibly be holy?" Because God is God, and He says because of the finished work at the Cross of Calvary all of your past, present, and future sin has been paid for. To avoid any misunderstanding, let's refer to Romans 6:1, which says, *Shall we go on sinning so that grace may increase?* Romans 6:2 answers this rhetorical question, *By no means!* The Bible teaches that grace is a gift offered freely to us, but it came at great expense to the Lord. We aren't peddling a "cheap grace gospel." We don't want to treat this precious gift with disrespect by abusing or misusing God's glorious plan for our lives. However, if we do step outside of God's will, are we cut off from His grace? No! As authentic believers in Christ, we are by God's mercy permanently under grace. Whether you are on the path of God's provision or the path of your performance, once in Christ, you remain under the canopy of God's grace.

We are forgiven. We are redeemed. We are holy.

Samantha, who released over thirty pounds, speaks to this: "I thought I was a slave to sin because that's how I felt every time I blew it, but Romans 6:14 says, 'For sin shall not be master over you, for you are not under law, but under grace.' I slowly began to see that it was my spiritual act of worship to surrender my body to God when I ate, to offer myself to Him as a living sacrifice. Day by day it became a sweet surrender."

Like Samantha, have you begun to discover the connection between eating and offering your body as a form of worship to a God who loves you? You may ask, "What happens when I 'blow it'? Is God grieved by my willful reluctance to surrender all unto Him or to my lack of faith to claim the power of the Holy Spirit?" He is grieved because we, as His beloveds, are missing out on His very best! But rest assured, you are forever His, and He will never break His blood covenant with you. His promises are eternally good and He is eternally faithful, even when we are not.

In light of these truths, what do *you* believe? Figure 14-2 shows the effect of believing that you are made new in Christ and that you are indeed holy.

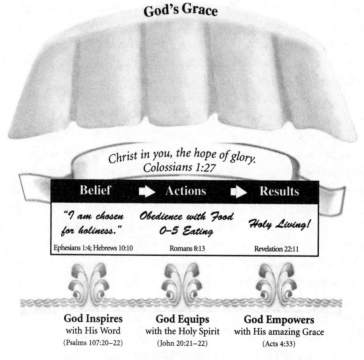

figure 14–2

Either we will be led by the Spirit, choosing to eat 0 to 5, or led by the flesh, where the mind remains fixated on food. By believing the Word of

God, that you are Holy in His sight, you will choose actions that are in line with that belief. You will be inspired, equipped, and empowered along the way by His grace and the Holy Spirit to choose in accordance with His will. Philippians 2:13 says, *For it is God who works in you to will and to act according to his good purpose.* This is walking on the path of God's provision.

Many of us may be confused about what an obedient life will look like. Beth Moore, Bible teacher and author, shares clearly, "Obedience does not mean sinlessness but confession and repentance when we sin. Obedience is not arriving at a perpetual state of godliness, but perpetually following hard after God. Obedience is not living miserably by a set of laws, but inviting the Spirit of God to flow freely through us so the power to be victorious comes from God and not from us. Obedience is learning to love and treasure God's Word and see it as our safety."[1]

Perhaps you are wondering, what is obedience where eating and food are concerned? Eating 0 to 5 is a practical way to put to death the deeds of the flesh. It is a holy action that will lead you to your natural God-given size. But remember that this will not make you righteous. As you seek His will to define what you are to believe about food, eating, and your body, here are some important safeguards:

+ **Be informed.**

The Bible is your primary resource for discovering God's truths regarding food, eating, and your body.

Continue to listen to your body's needs and pay more attention to 0 to 5 eating. Listen more closely to your body's cues regarding your reactions to particular foods. Do certain foods tempt you to binge later? Maybe that particular food or beverage could be released for a season into the hands of the Lord.

Rebecca found that coffee was her way of getting a jump-start on the day. However, as time went on, her coffee consumption increased by leaps and bounds. One day she decided that coffee had become a spiritual stronghold, and she needed a "coffee break," so she released it to the Lord. Now she has an occasional cup and enjoys it to the utmost, but coffee is no longer her lifeline.

You may also want to learn about general nutritional makeup of various foods. This need not become a preoccupation with reading food labels, but simply a way to be informed. As you are breaking free from food laws, remember you are free to be led by the Holy Spirit in what, when, and how much you eat. You will find your food choices will change and your selections will become wiser and healthier as you progress on the path of God's provision.

We also recommend that you remain flexible. For instance, today you may consider bacon and eggs to be your perfect breakfast and you feel energized after eating it. Yet, if ever you don't enjoy it as much or it begins to be disagreeable in some way, be creative and make a change. If you want to have an enchilada for breakfast, go for it. Be creative. Remember you are free to eat what you enjoy.

+ **Be willing.**

How are you feeling with regard to food at this point? If God were to make it clear that He wanted you to give up even more food, would you be willing to do so? Are you willing to share your food with others? Are you willing to cut your food in half portions?

Rebecca, a Thin Within participant who continues to release weight, writes, "I've had to accept the fact that I have a low metabolism and my body requires very little food. It's been painful but enlightening to realize that I don't need to eat three full meals a day."

As part of her maturing process, Rebecca had to be willing to hear God's voice and not insist on her "right" to three meals a day. It can be very challenging to break away from old beliefs, walk in the newness of the Spirit within and be obedient to the call of Christ. However, it is a challenge we must be willing to meet if we are to experience the abundant blessings of peace and joy that come from the Spirit-led life. Once Rebecca believed that God's grace was sufficient—even when she longed to eat more—she began to release weight and was well on the way to becoming her natural God-given size.

+ **Be faithful.**

Romans 14:23 says, "Everything that does not come from faith is sin." Being Spirit-led gives us the freedom to develop sensitivity and experience joy in listening to His voice moment by moment There is peace in knowing who we are in Christ, and there is confidence and rest for our souls when we surrender our will to a holy God.

This is what the LORD says: "Stand at the crossroads and look; ask for the ancient paths, ask where the good way is, and walk in it, and you will find rest for your souls" (Jeremiah 6:16).

As you offer your body as a living sacrifice and practice 0 to 5 eating, the

Lord will reveal His perfect will for you (Romans 12:2). As you surrender to His love, His transforming power of grace, and His provision, you will continue walking in the Spirit, down the path of God's provision.

Take Action

Choose to believe what God says about you as being holy and dearly beloved. Know that He desires you to be your natural God-given size. If you remain unconvinced, you will remain stuck in actions that go along with those negative beliefs. This is depicted in figure 14-3.

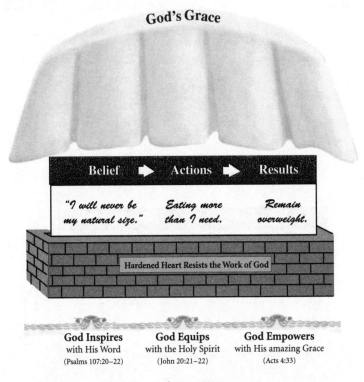

God's Grace

Belief	➡	Actions	➡	Results
"I will never be my natural size."		*Eating more than I need.*		*Remain overweight.*

Hardened Heart Resists the Work of God

God Inspires	God Equips	God Empowers
with His Word	with the Holy Spirit	with His amazing Grace
(Psalms 107:20–22)	(John 20:21–22)	(Acts 4:33)

figure 14–3

The conviction of the Holy Spirit reminds us that there are flesh-filled or faith-filled choices. To ignore this doesn't take us out from under the provision of God's grace, but it does numb us to the conviction of the Spirit. It is essential that our hearts remain tender and receptive to the leading of the Lord so that we come to full maturity (James 1:4).

God continues to offer inspiration through His Word, equipping through His Spirit, and empowering by His amazing grace. Hardened hearts cause our receptivity to these blessings to be muted or even completely calloused. If we allow this to happen, we will continue to believe lies and our actions will lead to disappointments and failure. This is not what God wants for His beloved!

What are some false beliefs or lies you have about *your* life? Your body? Your eating? Ask God to reveal these to you and record in the space below anything that has been hindering your actions and preventing holy results.

_____

_____

_____

_____

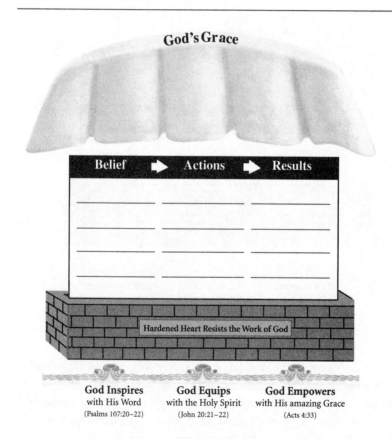

figure 14–4

Select four beliefs from your list, and place it in figure 14-4. Then fill in the actions that follow as a natural progression of that belief. What are the predictable results?

Are you content with these results? Do they line up with the goals that you established on Day Three? Is there something the Spirit is calling you to confess to God in prayer? If so, please do it now.

Replacing False Beliefs with Truth

Now that you have identified some false beliefs or lies that may hinder your progress, replace them with more beneficial truths from the Word of God.

Please read the following list from author, Dr. Neil Anderson:

1. Why should I say I can't, when the Bible says I can do all things through Christ who gives me strength? (Philippians 4:13)
2. Why should I lack, when I know that God shall supply all my needs according to His riches in glory in Christ Jesus? (Philippians 4:19)
3. Why should I fear, when the Bible says God has not given me a spirit of fear, but of power, love, and a sound mind? (2 Timothy 1:7)
4. Why should I lack faith to fulfill my calling, knowing that God has allotted to me a measure of faith? (Romans 12:3)
5. Why should I be weak, when the Bible says that the Lord is the strength of my life and that I will display strength and take action because I know God? (Psalm 27:1; Daniel 11:32)
6. Why should I allow Satan supremacy over my life, when He that is in me is greater than he that is in the world? (1 John 4:4)
7. Why should I accept defeat, when the Bible says that God always leads me in triumph? (2 Corinthians 2:14)
8. Why should I lack wisdom, when God generously gives wisdom to me when I ask Him for it? (1 Corinthians 1:30; James 1:5)
9. Why should I be depressed, when I can have hope by calling to mind God's loving-kindness, compassion, and faithfulness? (Lamentations 3:21–23)
10. Why should I ever be in bondage, knowing that there is liberty in the Spirit of the Lord? (Galatians 5:1)[2]

Enter one of these ten statements in figure 14-5. If you believe what God says in His word, what are some actions that will follow and what results will occur?

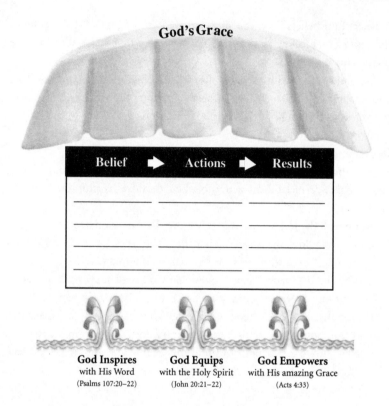

figure 14–5

The next time you face the pantry, refrigerator, or cookie jar, and you're really not hungry, ask yourself what you believe about your quest to become a vibrant, healthy temple of God. Ask yourself (and the Lord) what actions would follow if you were to believe what God's Word of truth says about you? God has promised to empower you so that your actions reap results that give glory to Him and an abiding joy within.

Your Success Story

Did you have any new insights while you were reading today? Please record them below.

_____

_____

_____

Verses to Ponder

But now he has reconciled you by Christ's physical body through death to present you holy in his sight, without blemish and free from accusation (Colossians 1:22).

Both the one who makes men holy and those who are made holy are of the same family. So Jesus is not ashamed to call them brothers (Hebrews 2:11).

For he chose us in him before the creation of the world to be holy and blameless in his sight (Ephesians 1:4).

Medical Moment

We firmly believe there are no "forbidden foods." However, it's important to say that *all foods are permissible, but not all foods are beneficial* (1 Corinthians 6:12). This truth is proven by the fact that the health of Americans has suffered severely because of poor eating habits. A recent USDA survey found that eighty-eight percent of children from ages six to eighteen have poor diets. Thirty years ago we spent one-third of our food dollars for food away from home. Today it is almost one-half, and food that is eaten out generally contains more saturated fat, less fiber, less calcium, and less iron. Each year Americans are eating over 150 pounds of sugar in the over-consumption of processed foods and beverages. Many people are unaware of the high sugar content in soft drinks, baked goods, cereals, pizza, bread, hot dogs, boxed rice mixes, crackers, spaghetti sauce, lunch meat, canned vegetables, flavored yogurt, ketchup, salad dressing, mayonnaise, and many kinds of peanut butter. The appropriate approach is not necessarily to eliminate all of the foods mentioned above. Instead, be informed of their content and allow God to lead you toward making wiser food choices.

As you apply the Thin Within principles and look to God and your body for signals as to which foods to choose, you will make healthier food choices. As you eat in this way, supplements shouldn't be necessary. However, since we are under grace, there is nothing wrong with taking an inexpensive multivitamin-mineral combination if you choose. Moderation is the key in food supplements as well.

—ARTHUR HALLIDAY, M.D.

Prayer

Dear Lord, thank You that as a believer in Christ I have a new Spirit within and that I can walk confidently under Your provision of amazing grace. I praise You, Lord, that Your grace is not conditional nor is it based on my performance but on Your provision. Help me to regard Your gift with gratitude and praise. I choose to believe You, Lord, and the truth of Your Word that You have given me power in Christ to tear down strong-holds—those things that have a strong hold on my thoughts and my actions. I look forward to the results that You are working out in me through Your Holy Spirit. In Jesus' name, Amen.

Success Tools

Tomorrow you will be preparing a special meal to be enjoyed using all of the keys to conscious eating. You may want to glance ahead to see how you can best prepare for tomorrow's activity.

+ Fill in the Thin Within Food Log.
+ Mark the Thin Within Observations and Corrections Chart for today.
+ Use the Thin Within Keys to Conscious Eating every time you choose to eat or drink today.

Thin Within Food Log

Hunger # before Eating	Time	Items/Amount	Hunger # after Eating

Thin Within Observations and Corrections Chart—Day 14

Observations	Day 14
1. I ate when my body was hungry.	
2. I ate in a calm environment by reducing distractions.	
3. I ate when I was sitting.	
4. I ate when my body and mind were relaxed.	
5. I ate and drank the things my body enjoyed.	
6. I paid attention to my food while eating.	
7. I ate slowly, savoring each bite.	
8. I stopped before my body was full.	

Thin Within Wisdom

Remember, whatever you believe affects your behavior and your behavior will determine your overall results. What will you believe today?

NOTES
1. Beth Moore, *Breaking Free Student Manual* (Nashville, Tennessee: LifeWay Press, 1999). Used by permission.
2. Neil T. Anderson, *Victory Over the Darkness* (Ventura, California: Regal Books, 1990), 115–117.

❧

Prevailing in the Pardon, Provision, Presence, and Power of God

Here I am! I stand at the door and knock.
If anyone hears my voice and opens the door,
I will come in and eat with him,
and he with me.
—Revelation 3:20

We have enjoyed delighting in the provision of God's amazing grace during these last few days. By knowing who we are and to whom we belong, we can walk in confidence by faith, led from within, by the Holy Spirit of God. We can bask in His presence and heed His voice as we surrender ourselves to Him.

Our faith is not to be relegated to church services on Sundays and perhaps Wednesday nights. Our faith is not a religion but a relationship with God, which involves breathing in His goodness and love, walking with Him, living each moment in conscious awareness that He is ever mindful of us.

What a blessing it is to be so loved by one who wants to be with us, even in the most mundane aspects of our lives. When we are faced with a crisis at work, we turn to Him. When a loved one falls ill, we turn to Him. When we don't know what to do next, we turn to Him. But how does God fit into our playtime? Does He accompany us on camping trips? Does He join us when we have lunch with our friends? What about quiet moments when we are driving? When we take the children to the park? When we relax in the bathtub with a good book?

Psalm 139 assures us that the Lord is with us no matter where we are. He wants us to make Him an *intentional* part of each moment of our lives through prayer. And how can we do this? It is as easy as breathing a prayer. As we open our eyes in the morning, "Good morning, Lord, and thank You for this new day."

As our children come through the door, "Thank You, Lord, for their health, their smiles, their love."

As we drive down the road, "Lord, please keep the drivers and pedestrians safe and give them a glimpse of You today."

As we sit down to a meal, "Lord, You have provided such a wonderful assortment of tastes. Thank You for Your bounty and creativity."

During the meal, "Lord, let this food provide me with strength to honor You."

As we reach our comfortable hunger level and stop at that 5, "Lord, I give back to You the rest of the food on my plate. Thank You for such abundance. I pray that others who lack might experience Your provisions."

The Lord longs for fellowship with each of us throughout our days and even those moments when we awaken at night. He is there. Breathing a prayer is easy and simple. Just a "Hello, Lord," touches His heart. Through informal conversations with Him we can walk with the Spirit and be continually renewed and refreshed by Him.

Jan Johnson, author and speaker, shares of her own experience developing a contemplative prayer life:

"As I experimented with unpretentious, plain-speaking conversation with God, the adventure began. God wasn't squinting down at me from His Supreme Court chair waiting to see if I mentioned every name on my [prayer] request list. He was sitting next to me on the backyard swing, eager to hear me, waiting me out, offering me cues."[1]

The Lord wants to have an ongoing conversation with us throughout the daily rhythms of our life. He is intimately acquainted with all of our ways. As we speak to Him, we acknowledge His presence and His involvement in our lives. This is what Paul means by praying continually (1 Thessalonians 5:17). Since our minds continue working all the time, our silent thoughts and prayers can constantly be offered to him in a running dialogue.

May my prayer be set before you like incense; may the lifting up of my hands be like the evening sacrifice (Psalm 141:2).

Even when Nehemiah was dialoguing with King Artaxerxes, he prayed a quick, silent "arrow" prayer to the Lord. In the same way, during our conversations with others we can remain aware of the presence of the Lord. If we allow ourselves to be conscious of His presence in the rhythms of life, we won't hesitate to include Him when we eat.

Today we are going to invite the Lord into a meal. Hopefully, you have come to find that eating from 0 to 5 is an enjoyable experience and that mealtime will become more of a time of communion between you and the

Lord. We are going to borrow from the familiar saying "today is the first day of the rest of your life" to direct you in planning and having "the very first meal of the rest of your life."

Everything about this meal will be absolutely intentional. Your focus will be on the Lord and on fostering an attitude of thankfulness during this meal experience.

Today you are going to have the pleasure of eating a meal *totally* in present time and in prayer. You are going to eat this meal as if eating were a new experience. Consider being totally conscious of every aspect of this meal, offering each minute of it to the Lord in worship and adoration of Him, His goodness to you, and His provision. The main purpose of this experience is to taste and see that the Lord is good.

On Day One, you answered questions about your last meal. You now have a recollection of how you used to eat compared with the Thin Within way of eating. For maximal enjoyment it's very important that you experience this particular meal at a 0. This meal will consist *only* of foods that delight you. It can be a meal that you prepare for yourself or one that is served to you. In either case please choose a favorite spot in which to eat.

The atmosphere is as important as the foods you choose. Try to create a calm environment without any distractions. Surround yourself with things that will enhance your eating experience. You might include your favorite china, music, silverware, flowers, special lighting. If you plan to eat in a restaurant, choose an ambiance that is pleasing as well. If you decide to have a picnic, select your favorite spot. It is best to eat this meal with the Lord as your only companion, although you may have someone with you if that person totally supports your desire to be conscious of your food and the Lord.

This meal is designed to be a pleasant experience, every bit of it enjoyed intentionally, consciously, and prayerfully as you savor the food.

Take Action
The First Meal of the Rest of Your Life

Read through the suggestions before starting, and then enjoy the meal!

1. Ask God to help you honor the body He has given you by maintaining the appropriate boundaries, including time and place. (We will discuss this more on Days Eighteen and Twenty-Five.) Reaffirm your love for Him and your desire to enjoy the food He has provided.

2. Select your favorite spot and wear clothes in which you are comfortable.

3. Check your hunger level. Plan to be at a 0 so that you can truly enjoy the food.

4. Take a moment to enter into God's presence as you invite Him to be a part of your dining experience.

5. Notice everything about the environment. No matter how familiar it may be, look at it as if you have never seen it before. Thank the Lord for all of His provisions.

6. Before you start eating, become aware of every item of food. Notice how it looks on the plate. Express your gratitude for the beauty in the colors of the food and its fragrance. Before taking your first bite, take a moment to thank God for His generous provisions, and pray that the food would bring physical satisfaction and health to your body.

7. Chew the food slowly and notice the different flavors and textures.

8. Sample each item and then ask yourself if it is enjoyable. Does it really delight you? Or did you just think it would?

9. How would you rate each item on your plate from 0 to 10 (0 being awful and 10 being terrific)?

10. Before you continue eating, check in with your hunger numbers. Stop eating when you're at a comfortable 5. Remember, your empty stomach is only as large as your *fist*.

11. When you've finished, once again thank and praise God, for this time and for what you have learned during the dining experience. Write down your observations about the meal.

_____

_____

_____

Observations about My Conscious Meal

In the chart below, evaluate which of the keys to conscious eating you applied during your "conscious meal." Was there something that kept you from applying one or more of the keys? In the middle column, simply write a "yes" or a "no." In the third column, record your thoughts about how that key affected your conscious eating experience.

Key	Did I use this key? Yes or No	Thoughts about how this key affected my meal experience
1. Eat only when my body is hungry.		
2. Reduce the number of distractions to eat in a calm environment		
3. Eat when I am sitting.		
4. Eat only when my mind and body are relaxed.		
5. Eat and drink the food and beverages that I enjoy.		
6. Pay attention to my food while eating.		
7. Eat slowly, savoring each bite.		
8. Stop before my body is full.		

✦ If you have any additional thoughts or observations about your conscious meal experience, jot them down in the space below.

_____

_____

_____

✦ Were you able to maintain 0 to 5 eating during this meal? Did you overeat?

_____

God is with us each and every moment of our lives. Eating, singing, walking, playing, driving, bathing, and working all can be joyful and worshipful experiences. Paul said whatever we do should be done to the glory of God, making Him known. As we do, we bring His love and delight to a darkened world that is so in need of Him. His presence makes us more sensitive to the needs of those around us, and helps us discover His love and His plan.

During your day take note if there are times when you seem isolated from His loving care and interest. Welcome Him in. He rejoices in that invitation and meets it gladly.

Your Success Story

Did you have any new insights while you were reading today? Please record them.

_____

_____

_____

Verses to Ponder

I pray that out of his glorious riches he may strengthen you with power through his Spirit in your inner being, so that Christ may dwell in your hearts through faith. And I pray that you, being rooted and established in love, may have power, together with all the saints, to grasp how wide and long and high and deep is the love of Christ, and to know this love that surpasses knowledge—that you may be filled to the measure of all the fullness of God (Ephesians 3:16–19).

Every day they continued to meet together in the temple courts. They broke bread in their homes and ate together with glad and sincere hearts (Acts 2:46).

Every good and perfect gift is from above, coming down from the Father of the heavenly lights, who does not change like shifting shadows (James 1:17).

Prayer

Dear Lord, thank You that I can savor Your goodness in the everyday things of life. You have given me the freedom to enjoy food and not to worry about what I will eat or drink or what I will wear. I pray, Lord, that I will remember that You are the provider of every good and perfect gift. Thank You for the fellowship that You provide and that I can delight in You, moment by moment. In Jesus' name, Amen.

Medical Moment

Most of my efforts as a practicing physician have been spent attempting to correct things that have been "broken." How much more rewarding it is, however, to focus on maintaining these wonderfully made bodies in proper working order and so to minimize the "breakdowns." How many times over the years has a patient said to me, "Why didn't I take better care of myself?" or "Why didn't I do something about this before I got sick?" Many of the conditions responsible for the most morbidity and mortality in this country—hypertension, heart disease, strokes, diabetes, and many degenerative and malignant disease—are either caused by or aggravated by our lifestyle habits. Some of the ills of humanity are beyond our control, but much human misery is man-made. We are each called to responsible stewardship for the gift of our bodies. Thin Within was developed and is offered to you to help you be a responsible and a faithful steward of your body, which is God's temple.

—ARTHUR HALLIDAY, M.D.

Success Tools

+ Continue keeping your food log, marking your hunger numbers.
+ Mark the Thin Within Observations and Corrections Chart.
+ Use the Thin Within Keys to Conscious Eating.

Thin Within Wisdom

The wonderful experience of your "perfect meal" can be recaptured each and every time you sit down to eat. Why not make the Lord a part of each meal today?

NOTE

1. Excerpted from *Enjoying the Presence of God* by Jan Johnson © 1996. Used by permission of NavPress Publishing Group. www.navpress.com. All rights reserved.

Thin Within Food Log

Hunger # before Eating	Time	Items/Amount	Hunger # after Eating

Thin Within Observations and Corrections Chart—Day 15

Observations	Day 15
1. I ate when my body was hungry.	
2. I ate in a calm environment by reducing distractions.	
3. I ate when I was sitting.	
4. I ate when my body and mind were relaxed.	
5. I ate and drank the things my body enjoyed.	
6. I paid attention to my food while eating.	
7. I ate slowly, savoring each bite.	
8. I stopped before my body was full.	

Victorious over Adversaries

Humble yourselves, therefore, under God's mighty hand,
that he may lift you up in due time.
Cast all your anxiety on him because he cares for you.
Be self-controlled and alert.
Your enemy the devil prowls around like a roaring lion
looking for someone to devour.
Resist him, standing firm in the faith.
—1 Peter 5:6–9a

The road we travel offers much adventure ahead as we continue on this path of God's provision. During the first phase of our journey we chose to submit our lives to God's loving grace. In doing so, you experienced His redemptive hand at work even in your trials and your failings. You learned how to use the observation and correction tool. This is your personal application of God's grace in the present moment, so that you can learn from your mistakes rather than pull out that "club of condemnation." You identified and discarded the old lies upon which you have built a faulty foundation, replacing them with the firm foundation of God's word.

As with most journeys of discovery we have been learning many things on the way, most recently that we can choose to build our lives according to God's specifications. As Moses and Solomon chose to believe and act on the instructions given by the Lord, we too will do the same. We observed on Day Fourteen how beliefs affect our actions, and our actions affect our results. If we want to live a holy life, we must believe what God says is true. He says we have been made new in Christ and that we are no longer slaves to sin. We are chosen for holiness. God also tells us that He continues to make us holy as we take our thoughts captive and submit them to the obedience of Christ.

Relying solely on God's grace, we experience His pardon, His provision, His presence, and His power as we follow Him. We invite God into every moment of our lives as we draw on the offering of His strength to walk in His Spirit. He inspires us through His word. He equips us by His Holy

Spirit. And He empowers us by His amazing grace to experience the results He desires.

Are you drawing more on His strength each moment, knowing that His grace is sufficient for your weakness? He is strong when you are weak. All of your trials and failures result in *godly* wisdom to guide you toward that which He intends for you and away from that which He does not when infused with the provision and power of the Holy Spirit. As you continue to allow Him to be the master and you the apprentice, you will delight in taking responsibility for the choices that exalt His plans and purposes.

We can now begin to see that the road ahead is less daunting than when we began. We have begun to release our hold on demanding our way, which doesn't have quite the appeal it did before we came to see Him as good, wise, and sovereign. We see that we have an opportunity to make choices that are in agreement with His divine purposes. In this there is peace and rest. He is our authority. He is our king. His ways are good. We begin to understand that the delight and peace found in submission is worth far more than "our rights," some of which we have relinquished.

As we submit ourselves to establishing godly goals and making choices that support realizing those goals, we will experience His success. But remember, we are people in process. God's destiny for you is to be free and to live up to your full potential in Christ Jesus. So, please persevere.

Look at your goals from Day Three. If you find that you are releasing some excess weight and that your pants are a bit looser, terrific. If you aren't, let's observe what is going on:

Problem: You still haven't experienced a reduction in size or weight.

Solution: Observe and correct.

Adjust your hunger numbers a bit. What you have called a 5 may be a 6. What you have called a 0 may actually be a 1 or a 2. That's all there is to it. No self-condemnation or wagging of fingers. No demerits. You can experience forgiveness, freedom, correction, and grace every step of the way. Tomorrow, we will introduce an effective tool that will help you even further. Remember: You are not a failure! You are God's beloved, so rise up and walk in His ways!

Evaluate your goal #1 from Day Three. Is it doable in the strength of the Lord? Do you believe that He is able to accomplish this in you? He doesn't want you to try to accomplish it in your own strength. That would take you back to the path of your performance. Take the goal to God in prayer right now. Ask Him if He wants you to adjust it. Do the same with goal #2 and goal #3 as well. Evaluate if they are, in fact, God's goals for you.

By now you are aware that we are called by God to live in present time (Matthew 6:25–34). At this moment, you can observe and correct. If you feel you are on track, then rewrite your goals in the space provided. Adjust them if God leads you to do so, keeping in mind that God loves to make your dreams in Him come true.

Date: _____

Goal #1: _____

Goal #2: _____

Goal #3: _____

Congratulations! Rather than live in defeat and "failure" over not realizing your goals from Day Three, you can observe and correct and begin again. Renew your commitment to give your all over the next fourteen days. Stand in agreement with God knowing that His goals for you are fulfilled by making godly choices. Remember that His grace was never intended to be merely a pardon for past, present, and future sins. His grace is also a provision for your daily, moment-by-moment needs. Invite Him to infuse your life, enabling you to have insight, wisdom, discernment, and power to live according to His best for you.

You have now observed that your resistance to eating only when you are truly hungry and to stop when you are comfortable has very little to do with the needs of your body. Many factors enter into the equation, such as thinking that your body is your own to do with as you please. Emotions also can trigger "fat machinery," which we will now refer to as "flesh machinery," reflecting the fact that when it is operative, we have chosen to follow the desires of the flesh rather than the Spirit.

We have seen that our flesh machinery can kick into gear in a variety of situations, such as going to lunch because it's twelve o'clock noon even when we're not hungry.

We are now going to look at situations or significant times in your life that can trigger flesh machinery and result in unconscious, automatic eating. We pray the Holy Spirit will give you discernment and allow God's grace, goodness, and sovereignty to minister to your soul. Invite Him to help you see clearly the events that may have contributed to your inappropriate eating. Jesus said in John 8:32, "*Then you will know the truth, and the truth will set you free.*"

This exercise may require some extra courage as you begin to identify and revisit some events or significant times of your life. Please know that God will use your life experiences to draw you closer to Him, to strengthen your faith, and to mold your character. Nothing is wasted in God's amazing economy. By bringing your past into the light, God's grace can restore and transform you.

My own experience of a "significant time" that impacted my life dramatically happened when I was twenty years old. I was going to school to become a hygienist. It was there I met a young man and I gave my heart to him. In my indiscretion, I became pregnant. Even though marriage was proposed, in my insecurity and selfishness I chose what appeared to be the easy way out. Not knowing God, but knowing my own feelings of panic, I determined to do what was right in my own eyes, which was to have an abortion. I was very ashamed, and I kept it a secret from my parents and from my friends. Abortions were illegal in this country at that time and after four and a half frantic months of searching, I finally found a contact in Tijuana, Mexico. I didn't speak Spanish and the people there didn't speak English, but I was desperate. By the grace of God, I didn't have any major physical repercussions, so after the abortion I thought I was fine. I assumed that what was done was done, and I could get on with life. But I wasn't fine, and I couldn't seem to get on with life.

I'm reminded of the passage from Proverbs 16:25 that says it so well: *There is a way that* seems *right to a man but in the end it leads to death* (emphasis added). The choice I made led to the sudden death of an unborn child and to the slow death in my own spirit and soul. I got mixed up with the wrong crowd and in a very fast-lane lifestyle of drugs and alcohol. I started bingeing and purging many times during a day. I gained thirty-eight pounds and sank into a deep pit of despair.

I would come home with shopping bags full of junk food, pull down the shades in my apartment, and stuff myself until I was sick or until I made myself vomit. Finally, not being able to face another day of self-loathing, I hit bottom. I remember as if it were yesterday, sitting on my couch in my dingy apartment with tears running down my face, ready to execute my plan to end my life.

Then a miraculous thing happened. God intervened. He literally reached down from on high and rescued me. As the psalmist says, *He lifted me out of the slimy pit, out of the mud and mire; he set my feet on a rock and gave me a firm place to stand* (Psalm 40:2). God took away the shame of my lascivious life. I was suddenly washed clean. My despair was turned to hope. I was overwhelmed with His presence, His mercy, and His grace.

God, whom I didn't even know and had even denied, gave me a new beginning, a second chance. I wish I could say I was miraculously saved at that time, but I guess I'm a slow learner. However, this did begin my search for the meaning of this supernatural experience and the purpose of my life, a quest that led me some twenty-two years later to the foot of the cross.

As you can see, significant past events, with or without our awareness, can affect the way we relate to food and our bodies.

Let's take a look at how significant events in your past may have affected the way you deal with food and your body. In this exercise ask God to shed His light on four events He wants to bring to mind as most significant or influential in your life. You may want to consider others at a later time. As you do this, we encourage you to focus on the face of Jesus. As we have seen in previous days, no failure, mistake, or sin is beyond God's ability to redeem. It is in this place that you can see just how much you need Him and just how capable He is to meet all your needs.

Significant Times Exercise

This exercise includes a list of seventeen events that may have influenced the way you relate to food, your body, and eating. If we have not listed an event of crucial importance for you, please add it. Pick four from the list and place them in order from the earliest incident to the most recent. Place each event in the proper spaces provided. An incident may appear on your list more than once.

1. First sexual encounter _____

2. Fell in love _____

3. Failed relationship _____

4. Sexual trauma_____

5. Moved away from home_____

6. New job _____

7. Married_____

8. Infidelity _____

9. Pregnancy_____

10. Abortion _____

11. Having or raising children _____

12. Got divorced or separated _____

13. Major illness (yours or another person's)_____

14. Lost job_____

15. Major relocation_____

16. Disappearance of someone close to you_____

17. Death of someone close to you _____

Take a moment now to circle or add to this list your four most influential times before you proceed with this exercise. Offer these significant events to God in prayer. Ask Him to prepare your mind and your heart for any godly truth He chooses to reveal about how these events have influenced your life. Then, focus individually on these four significant times and notice what the Holy Spirit brings to your attention.

Significant Time #1

Where were you? _____

Who was with you? _____

How did you feel? _____

Was there a shift in your weight as a result of this incident? _____

What decisions did you make as a result of this incident? _____

Did your self-esteem increase or decrease? _____

How did this incident affect your view of God? _____

Significant Time #2

Where were you? _____

Who was with you? _____

How did you feel? _____

Was there a shift in your weight as a result of this incident? _____

What decisions did you make as a result of this incident? _____

Did your self-esteem increase or decrease? _____

How did this incident affect your view of God? _____

Significant Time #3

Where were you? _____

Who was with you? _____

How did you feel? _____

Was there a shift in your weight as a result of this incident? _____

What decisions did you make as a result of this incident? _____

Did your self-esteem increase or decrease? _____

How did this incident affect your view of God? _____

Significant Time #4

Where were you? _____

Who was with you? _____

How did you feel? _____

Was there a shift in your weight as a result of this incident? _____

What decisions did you make as a result of this incident? _____

Did your self-esteem increase or decrease? _____

How did this incident affect your view of God? _____

Now go back and prayerfully reread your answers. Did you "lose" or "gain" weight as a result of the situation? How did you feel about your body as a result of any of these events? These are examples of a more subtle form of flesh machinery. Take captive these thoughts and offer them to your Savior and Lord. We understand that it may be very challenging to face these significant events in your life. Please keep in mind that the love of our Lord is ever present with you, and He will restore and redeem each one of them. Consider the following question asked by Brennan Manning: "Do you really accept the message that God is head over heels in love with you? I believe that this question is at the core of our ability to mature and grow spiritually. If in our hearts we really don't believe that God loves us as we are, if we are still tainted by the lie that we can do something to make God love us more, we are rejecting the message of the cross."[1]

You are loved just as you are, regardless of your past or your role in it. No matter what shame you may feel, you are precious to God, who is "head over heels in love with you."

Perhaps you can identify with Amanda, a Thin Within participant. She explains, "As I considered allowing myself to get hungry—really truly absolutely stomach hungry—I was terrified! Whenever I got hungry, I would panic! I asked God to show me why. He revealed to me that I was fearful because much of the abuse I experienced as a child involved the dinner table, food, and what I would or wouldn't eat. I had terrible memories associated with food." It was very difficult, but as Amanda faced her past in the light of God's truth, she began to see that she could hold the hand of God as she waited to reach her 0. With that insight, the healing process could begin as she learned to eat in present time. She continues by saying, "The Lord met me in that place of absolute need and vulnerability. It was there that I could cuddle up onto His lap and experience His soothing love for me. The 'big bad woman' that was my mother no longer followed me into every hunger pang or meal. I began to see 0 as a place of growth and maturity. It wasn't easy, but our God is able."

[God] *is able to do far more abundantly beyond all that we ask or think* (Ephesians 3:20, NASB).

Take Action

+ Evaluate your own eating. Do so with grace and compassion. Do you find that you are fearful of 0? Are you eating based on body hunger or heart hunger? Are you seeking to satisfy an insatiable appetite? Have you been misreading your body's cues? Record your observations and comments.

_____

_____

Let's ask ourselves once again, what does the past have to do with the present or present-time eating? And the answer is absolutely nothing! Present-time eating is asking your body if it is hungry and eating the foods you enjoy now from 0 to 5 or less.

Like Amanda, we too can take hold of God's hand and experience His grace and healing. He will turn even painful things to purposeful things—in fact He is glorified in doing so. Pray that God will help you to see your past as He sees it—as redeemable. It is so comforting to know that God does not waste anything in our lives. He uses everything to shape and mold us into His likeness.

In order to live and eat in the present time, after my abortion and battle with bulimia, I forgave those involved and myself. Ultimately with God's grace, I was able to bless that painful time, to let it go and move on. Without that experience and the subsequent struggle, I would not be writing this book to you, dear readers. You, too, can choose to release the past and allow God to continue the restorative work He has begun in your life.

Your Success Story

Did you have any new feelings or ideas while you were reading today? Please record them below.

_____

_____

_____

Verses to Ponder

The LORD upholds all those who fall and lifts up all who are bowed down. The eyes of all look to you, and you give them their food at the proper time. You open your hand and satisfy the desires of every living thing. The LORD is righteous in all his ways and loving toward all he has made. The LORD is near to all who call on him, to all who call on him in truth (Psalm 145:14–18).

Yet I am always with you; you hold me by my right hand. You guide me with your counsel, and afterward you will take me into glory. Whom have I in heaven but you? And earth has nothing I desire besides you (Psalm 73:23–25).

Prayer

Dear God, please help me to be honest with You and with myself and not to allow my past to dictate my behavior in present time. I want to see myself as You see me—as holy and beloved in Your eyes—and to know that You are able to work for "good" in those things that I may see as "bad" or "ugly." Help me to use food as You intended rather than to misuse it to stuff down my feelings. Sometimes it is hard for me to tell the difference. But I turn to You, Lord, and allow You to quiet my mind as I pray for godly discernment and healing. In Jesus' name, Amen.

Medical Moment

We can deal with the trauma of our past in one of three ways:

1. By denial—never accepting on a conscious level that we were hurt or wounded by someone or something ("no one ever abused me").

2. By staying stuck in it—acknowledging that something bad happened but hanging on to it as an excuse for whatever goes wrong in our lives ("I'm the way I am because I was abused, and I'll never be any better").

3. By appropriating it as part of our growth (even though painful) in a fallen world and letting it strengthen us to face the trials and tribulations of the future ("I was abused, but by overcoming it with the Lord, the truth of His Word, and forgiveness, I'm a stronger person now").

God's ultimate goal for us is to bind up the broken-hearted, freeing all from the tyranny of the past, to experience joy, peace, and love in the present.

—ARTHUR HALLIDAY, M.D.

Success Tools

+ Fill in the Thin Within Food Log.
+ Mark the Thin Within Observations and Corrections Chart for today.
+ Use the Thin Within Keys to Conscious Eating every time you choose to eat or drink today.

Thin Within Food Log

Hunger # before Eating	Time	Items/Amount	Hunger # after Eating

Thin Within Observations and Corrections Chart—Day 16

Observations	Day 16
1. I ate when my body was hungry.	
2. I ate in a calm environment by reducing distractions.	
3. I ate when I was sitting.	
4. I ate when my body and mind were relaxed.	
5. I ate and drank the things my body enjoyed.	
6. I paid attention to my food while eating.	
7. I ate slowly, savoring each bite.	
8. I stopped before my body was full.	

Thin Within Wisdom

When it seems difficult to face the past, reach for the hand of your Savior. He will walk with you through the Valley of the Shadow and get you through to the other side.

NOTE

1. Brennan Manning, *The Ragamuffin Gospel* (Sisters, Oregon: Multnomah Press, 2000), 159.

The Grandeur of Gratitude

Give thanks in all circumstances,
for this is God's will for you in Christ Jesus.
—1 Thessalonians 5:18

With thankful hearts we enjoy the pardon, power, presence, and provision of our God and king who is with us constantly. During Day Fifteen you were encouraged to invite the Lord into your meal experience as He infused even the mundane with His joy, His peace, His power, and His love.

Yesterday we discovered how significant past events can affect the present moment. We urged you to remain conscious of this in your approach to food and your body.

If the truths we have been sharing with you have been challenging, we understand and ask you to turn your eyes toward Him and allow the Holy Spirit to minister to your soul (John 14:26).

It was *before* you "got it all together" that Jesus gave His life for you (Romans 5:8). He ordained that you would belong to Him before the creation of the earth (Ephesians 1:4). Even when your mistakes were on his shoulders, your shame weighing on his mind, even then He chose to love you (Luke 23:34).

No matter what, you can climb up into your Heavenly Abba's lap and listen to Him sing to you with delight (Zephaniah 3:17). In Isaiah 40:11, we are told that He tends us like a shepherd and that He gathers us to his chest in an affirmation of His tender love. Rest in His embrace.

With so great a saving grace, with so unfathomable a love, with so tender a mercy, *what, then, shall we say in response to this* (Romans 8:31)? We can only stand in humble awe and amazement.

This is the one to whom we bow.

This is the one we worship.

This is the one to whom we offer our praise and our thanks.

Do not be anxious about anything, but in everything, by prayer and petition, with thanksgiving, present your requests to God. And the peace of God, which transcends all understanding, will guard your hearts and your minds in Christ Jesus (Philippians 4:6–7).

As we turn to Him, offering up our prayers and petitions with thankful hearts, God's peace stands guard. As we bow in humble gratitude for all He has done for us, we begin to see that His peace, beyond our ability to fathom, permeates us through and through. This peace stands as a sentry guarding our hearts and minds. As we acknowledge that He is the sovereign God and that we are His precious chosen children, we are lifted on high and are able to see from His vantage point. This place of humility has the greatest view.

Humble yourselves before the Lord, and he will lift you up (James 4:10).

From here we are able to see our shortcomings as opportunities for God to demonstrate His sovereign power. We see our trials as occasions to exercise faith as we wait on God's answer. We see Him as sovereign and in supreme authority, yet intimately involved with everything. In this place of gratitude, we are able to rest and surrender to His plan, His will, His spirit, His power, and His presence.

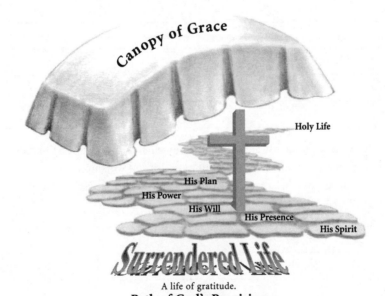

A life of gratitude.
Path of God's Provision
Two Steps Forward and One Back • Heading Toward the Holy Life • Confidence in God

figure 17–1

Come, let us bow down in worship, let us kneel before the LORD our Maker; for he is our God and we are the people of his pasture, the flock under his care (Psalm 95:6–7).

It is with a heart of gratitude that we live the surrendered life as is illustrated in fig. 17-1.

Take Action

Gratitude Giving—An Exercise in Thankfulness

Prayerfully ask the Lord to reveal to you all the things for which you are thankful. Reflect back on all that has occurred over the past sixteen days. Nothing is too small to be acknowledged. Record each blessing below.

_____

_____

_____

_____

_____

_____

_____

_____

_____

_____

Now reread your list and imagine yourself standing before Him. Offer these things and your thanks to Him as praise and worship.

Jot down your insights after you have done this exercise. How do you feel? Why?

_____

_____

_____

As we continue to be thankful to the Lord, we discover that the shackles of self-preoccupation and greed begin to fall away, that our incessant need or want for more food begins to diminish. We discover that we are being transformed from within. It is in this place of continued surrender that we lay before Him our hearts, our hunger, and, yes, our food. We are so grateful for the body He has given us and for His daily provisions. His grace and mercy are measureless.

An attitude of gratitude will strengthen you on the next exciting leg of our journey. The following is another tool to use, *if you choose*, for the remainder of this trek. It is designed to assist you to be as honest as possible with yourself in your food and eating habits. It is not designed to be a justification for self-glorification or self-condemnation. It is offered as another tool for observation and correction.

Hunger Graph

This is one of the most effective tools to help you become even more familiar with your hunger levels and eating patterns. A good tool becomes transparent over time, which means that after using it for a while you don't even notice it, and this will happen for you in using the hunger graph, so that by the end of our thirty days together it will be internalized. By then, you'll just naturally wait until you feel hungry before eating and you'll stop at the proper point because your body and the Spirit within will say "enough." In fact, please only use this hunger graph *if you feel the need for additional support and accountability.*

To use this graph, record the time of day and your hunger numbers before and after eating. The example shows how the graph would look if you ate from a 1 to a 6 at 11 A.M., from a 0 to a 5 at 5 P.M., and from a 2 to a 5 at midnight. The diagonal lines show times between eating and diminishing fullness. Each time you choose to eat or drink anything other than water during the twenty-four-hour period, record the time along with your "before" and "after" hunger numbers.

Suppose in reflecting on your hunger graphs at the end of the week, you see that at your daily 11 A.M. coffee break you tend to start eating when you're not at a 0 and you go above a 5. Why? What is going on at that time that causes you to overeat? Maybe you overate because your friends asked you to go on a meal break, maybe because you were weary and frustrated, or perhaps it was because of willful rebellion. Whatever you observe, there's a likelihood of eating above a 5 because you didn't start at a 0. So observe the patterns from your hunger graph and put in the appropriate corrections.

Look for creative options. Maybe you'll choose not to eat at midnight (see the graph) so you'll truly be at a 0 the next morning. You may even choose to remain at 0 until 11 A.M. so you can really enjoy your meal break with your friends.

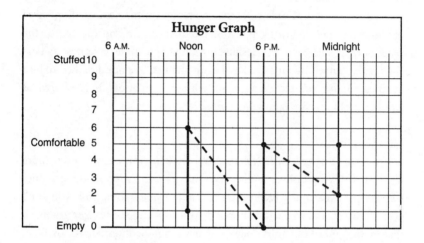

Jeanette, who released twenty pounds in just six weeks said, "At first I was nervous about using the hunger graph. I was trying to break free of my compulsive use of charts and devices to evaluate my progress and myself. But I felt as if the Lord was encouraging me to give it a try and as I began to use it, I found grace there. Even though I observed that I started eating when I was at a 1 rather than a 0, I felt so relieved because that was real progress for me.

"I also discovered some interesting habits that I hadn't realized previously. I noticed that each day at about 3 P.M. I would start eating when I wasn't even hungry. I was actually about a 3 on the hunger scale, and invariably I would end up over my comfortable 5. Then for the rest of the day I would nibble and not let myself get close to 0 for the rest of the day."

Jeanette continued, "I decided to spend some additional time with the Lord in prayer each day just before eating and I also tried to be more aware of my emotions during the afternoon and evening. It worked. After a couple of weeks my hunger numbers were more reflective of 0 to 5 eating. By observing and correcting, my mid-afternoon slide downhill had been halted."

If you choose to use it, we hope you find the hunger graph as helpful as Jeanette. It actually serves three purposes.

1. It provides an excellent visualization of your eating patterns.
2. It ties your hunger numbers to time. This allows you to see what isn't working for you and then prayerfully put in the appropriate correction.
3. It is an excellent way for you to see if you're eating because of true body hunger or for some other reason.

This tool can be used by God to help you walk with greater integrity so that each step of the way you are maturing in your walk with the Lord. As a result, you will be pleased, and God will be honored.

As you choose to honor Him with your choices regarding food and eating, you will continue to experience the blessing of releasing weight down to your natural God-given size. God is mighty. God is willing to perform this work in you which gives you cause to pause and offer gratitude!

Your Success Story

Did you have any new insights while you were reading today? Please record them below.

_____

_____

_____

Verses to Ponder

I will give thanks to the LORD because of his righteousness and will sing praise to the name of the LORD Most High (Psalm 7:17).

The LORD is my strength and my shield; my heart trusts in him, and I am helped. My heart leaps for joy and I will give thanks to him in song (Psalm 28:7).

Enter his gates with thanksgiving and his courts with praise; give thanks to him and praise his name. For the LORD is good and his love endures for ever; his faithfulness continues through all generations (Psalm 100:4–5).

The LORD will surely comfort Zion and will look with compassion on all her ruins; he will make her deserts like Eden, her wastelands like the garden of the LORD. Joy and gladness will be found in her, thanksgiving and the sound of singing (Isaiah 51:3).

Medical Moment

The human body never ceases to amaze me—thousands of functions communicating and interconnecting between dozens of complex operating systems. And one of the most incredible aspects of the entire system is how God designed the steady supply of fuel (sugar) that each cell needs for optimal functioning. The food we ingest is broken down into absorbable components—fatty acids from fats, amino acids from proteins, and simple sugar from complex carbohydrates. Sugar is either used immediately, stored in the liver as glycogen, or converted to fats for future use if the food supply is insufficient. When there is no immediate supply of sugar, the liver glycogen is released into the blood, and when that source is depleted, energy is released from our fat deposits. (There is a one- or two-day supply of energy in each pound of fat.) Two questions frequently arise in connection with sugar—hypoglycemia and sugar addiction.

Hypoglycemia (low blood sugar) has been popularized in the lay press as causing a variety of common symptoms such as fatigue, nervousness, headache, and hunger. While hypoglycemia can occur, it is extremely uncommon and can be accurately established only by a blood test. Most of the symptoms ascribed to hypoglycemia are precipitated by other events, not low blood sugar. As for sugar addiction, some people experience an intense craving for sweets, difficulty stopping eating sweets and a variety of symptoms when sweets are not available. Sugar may be to those people what is called a "trigger food." Blood sugar levels do apparently raise the level of serotonin in the brain, which may be the mechanism for these situations, but it isn't a true addiction in the sense that there are no withdrawal symptoms (as in alcoholism) when sugar is not eaten.

—Arthur Halliday, M.D.

Prayer

Lord, please fill my heart with thanksgiving. I want to praise You and thank You for what You are doing in my body, mind, and spirit. Sometimes I get so fixed on what I want instead of all You have done for me that I lose sight of what a gracious and merciful God You are. Please redirect my focus, Lord. Cause me to rejoice in all You have provided and the fact that You desire to have fellowship with me at each and every moment. Thank You for Your restorative work on my body, inside and out! I praise You, as I know that Your works are wonderful. In Your precious name I pray, Amen.

Success Tools

+ Fill in your hunger graph today, if you choose, marking in your hunger levels and connecting the dots so you can observe your eating patterns. You might make a copy of this graph and carry it with you, as it is easy to forget how much we eat during a busy day. Remember too that if you mark down one number (say a 5) and twenty minutes later you feel like you've eaten to a 7, then go back and correct your numbers—because the last reading is the accurate reading.
+ Fill in the Thin Within Food Log.
+ Mark the Thin Within Observations and Corrections Chart for today.
+ Use the Thin Within Keys to Conscious Eating when you choose to eat or drink today.

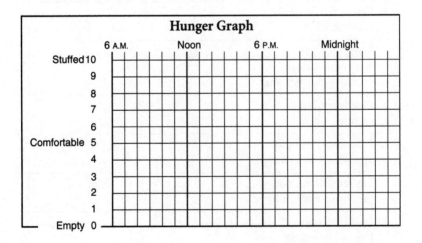

Thin Within Food Log

Hunger # before Eating	Time	Items/Amount	Hunger # after Eating

Thin Within Observations and Corrections Chart—Day 17

Observations	Day 17
1. I ate when my body was hungry.	
2. I ate in a calm environment by reducing distractions.	
3. I ate when I was sitting.	
4. I ate when my body and mind were relaxed.	
5. I ate and drank the things my body enjoyed.	
6. I paid attention to my food while eating.	
7. I ate slowly, savoring each bite.	
8. I stopped before my body was full.	

Thin Within Wisdom

The place of humility has the greatest view.

From there we are able to see our shortcomings as opportunities for God to demonstrate His sovereign power.

❧

Bringing Honor to the Temple— Building Godly Boundaries

*LORD, you have assigned me my portion and my cup;
You have made my lot secure.
The boundary lines have fallen for me in pleasant places;
surely I have a delightful inheritance.*
—Psalm 16:5–6

One of the wonderful aspects about our Thin Within journey is that we can enjoy any food that God has made. Truly our boundary lines have fallen in pleasant places. No food is unclean. No food is "bad." There is joy and freedom found in approaching food this way. Listening to your body and eating between 0 and 5 is a rewarding experience. As you apply the keys to conscious eating, your extra weight really will begin to melt away.

On our journey we have focused on the rebuilding and restoring process that God desires for your body, His temple. Just as taking a long walk can strengthen the physical body, so too this spiritual "walk" or journey will be strengthening. As Paul says in 1 Timothy 4:8, *Physical training is of some value, but godliness has value for all things, holding promise for both the present life and the life to come.*

As we journey, we discover that not only are we being built up in mind, body, spirit, and soul, we are building godly lives that have promise now and for eternity.

We will focus today on the biblical principle of establishing and maintaining godly boundaries. We have already begun to give time and attention, to certain aspects of boundary setting over the past seventeen days. It is the call of God to each one of us to protect the body He has given to us, to treat it well, to use it to serve Him, and to listen to His voice in the process.

What is our most basic boundary? It is, of course, our body. We determine what enters in and what stays out. But before we consider specific boundaries, let's reflect on boundaries in general.

Many opportunities in which to invest our time, attention, and energy beckon us. We have to decide which ones God wants us to pursue. It is often difficult for us to reject opportunities, even if the Lord leads us to say "no." Likewise, at times we experience difficulty saying "yes" when He leads us to say "yes." Still, we have the freedom to determine how and to whom we will allocate our time, treasures, and talents. It is important, then, that we seek God's perspective on this topic and to carefully obey His call.

To investigate what the Scriptures teach about godly boundaries, we first turn to Nehemiah who led God's people to rebuild the walls around Jerusalem following the return of the exiles from Babylon. What others couldn't accomplish in decades, this man led the Israelites to complete in just fifty-two days. Much of his success was due to the fact that he had a clear understanding, a respect for, and an adherence to godly boundaries.

The book of Nehemiah records that two influential men named Sanballat and Tobiah were determined to prevent Jerusalem's walls from being built. Their determination ran counter to the purposes of Nehemiah and God. Initially, Sanballat and Tobiah were merely disturbed by the plans the Israelites had for the walls. Then, as time passed, these prominent men begin to verbally mock and ridicule God's people. However, Nehemiah remained focused on the boundaries that had been established by the Lord:

I answered them by saying, "The God of heaven will give us success. We his servants will start rebuilding, but as for you, you have no share in Jerusalem or any claim or historic right to it" (Nehemiah 2:20).

When their strategy of mocking didn't work, Sanballat tried to bait soldiers to attack the workers. When that didn't work, he planned a frontal assault.

They all plotted together to come and fight against Jerusalem and stir up trouble against it. But we prayed to our God and posted a guard day and night to meet this threat (Nehemiah 4:8–9).

God continued to answer the prayers of His people, and the assault strategy failed. Sanballat then took the "sweet as honey" approach and tried to lure Nehemiah into a trap. Nehemiah, however, knew what his enemies were up to. Committed to the work of God, he declared, *I am carrying on a great project and cannot go down. Why should the work stop while I leave it and go down to you?* (Nehemiah 6:3)

Nehemiah wasn't about to be derailed by an ungodly alliance. Thus far, no spears, swords, or arrows had actually been used; the only weapons had been words. But Nehemiah remained resolute, guarding his life, as well as his God-given calling and work from the evil intentions of others. And he encouraged the people entrusted to his care to do the same.

When the final plot was underway to lure Nehemiah into the temple of God and to manipulate him into breaking the law, he remained faithful to God's boundaries. Nehemiah refused to sin against the Lord and remained steadfast in his life of obedience to God. This account demonstrates that godly boundaries can be established and maintained in a God-honoring way. As a result, Nehemiah is recorded in biblical history as one of the great men of all time.

Jesus also established and protected His God-given boundaries. The first two chapters of the book of Mark tell us that after an intense day of ministry, which included exorcising a demon, preaching to multitudes, and healing crowds of people until well after sunset, Jesus still maintained boundaries regarding how He would spend His time. No doubt He was exhausted by his rigorous schedule, yet He arose early to meet with His Father:

Very early in the morning, while it was still dark, Jesus got up, left the house and went off to a solitary place, where he prayed (Mark 1:35).

Jesus pulled away from people, even from his close friends, because He knew of the power available in the presence of the Father.

Simon and his companions went to look for him, and when they found him, they exclaimed: "Everyone is looking for you!" Jesus replied, "Let us go somewhere else—to the nearby villages—so I can preach there also. That is why I have come" (Mark 1:36–38).

Some of those looking for Jesus were probably people He had ministered to on the previous night. Perhaps they'd brought along others who longed to experience His healing touch as well. However, we see that even in this case where many needs were left unmet, where many still longed for Jesus' time, attention, and energy, He set a godly boundary and He maintained it.

As we seek to establish and maintain godly boundaries, we need to understand there will always be people placing more and different demands upon us than God does. It is our responsibility to guard our minds, spirits, hearts, and bodies from people who bombard us with distractions and who may draw us to less-than-godly purposes.

Regina has released eighty pounds and is well on her way to her natural God-given size. She said, "I thought I could never say no to any request made of me, even if everything in me knew I shouldn't do it. I thought that by seeking to please everyone else, I would be more acceptable. But I observed when I was overcommitted, I would stuff myself with food. Then I wasn't able to listen to the voice of the Holy Spirit and honor my own needs. I am learning to think and pray about a commitment before I jump in and now sometimes I say 'no.'"

We can learn to avoid the trap of "finding a need and filling it" simply by being still and knowing that God doesn't call us to be all things to all people. This is modeled throughout the Scriptures. In our desire for human approval and not wanting to offend others by saying "no," we may deplete the energy we need for going about the Father's business. On the other hand, with proper boundaries we become energized in ministering to others and in service of our Lord.

It is possible that those significant events you reviewed on Day Sixteen may affect your ability to establish godly boundaries. For example, if others have treated you inappropriately and violated your personal boundaries, you may not have a clear understanding as to what makes boundaries godly and what makes them inappropriate. If so, it is especially important for you to seek the Lord, and possibly godly counsel, to determine what appropriate boundaries are for you at this time. What a wonderful opportunity this can be for maturity in the Lord. As our restoration work continues, let's remain aware of ways in which the enemy has encroached on us in the past, so we can be better prepared in the future.

"Everything is permissible for me"—but not everything is beneficial. "Everything is permissible for me"—but I will not be mastered by anything (1 Corinthians 6:12).

Nothing and no one should master us but Christ. We have the freedom to enjoy many delightful things, yet we need never again accept the constraints of obligation or obsession. As we establish and maintain godly boundaries, we may discover something new. We begin to respond in the Spirit rather than to react in the flesh.

One way we can apply this to our Thin Within journey is in our choice of food. Which foods will you choose for your 0 to 5 eating experience? Since you have permission to enjoy all things but refuse to be mastered by anything, you can evaluate the foods and place them into categories—and we don't mean fats, carbohydrates, and protein!

The first category is called "pleasers." They have some very desirable qualities, which are described as follows:

Pleasers

1. You think of the food without or before seeing it. It is something you know you will enjoy.
2. You desire it from deep down. When you are at a 0, you know that this is a food that will hit the spot and bring physical satisfaction.
3. The food may not be readily available. It might be offered only at favorite restaurant or prepared by someone special. It may even be necessary for you to prepare it in your own kitchen. It's the sort of food for which you would walk a mile, and it is totally satisfying when you do get it.
4. Pleasers are very specific. For instance, not "generic" chocolate, but Godiva chocolate. Not just any pizza, but thin-crust Thai pizza with a special kick to the sauce. Not just any spinach salad, but one that has onions, artichoke hearts, fresh tomatoes, and a yummy balsamic vinegar dressing on it. (You can tell that's a pleaser for me.)
5. Pleasers may change from day to day. It may take practice and patience to discover your true pleasers. Be adventuresome and have fun in the process.

Maybe you're wondering if the notion of a pleaser is biblical. We think it is. There are references to "choice food" in the Scriptures. For example,

Nehemiah said, "Go and enjoy choice food and sweet drinks, and send some to those who have nothing prepared. This day is sacred to our Lord. Do not grieve, for the joy of the LORD is your strength" (Nehemiah 8:10).

We recommend discovering your pleasers and allowing those foods to be the ones on which you "spend" your 0 to 5 eating. The Bible indicates the Lord is pleased when we delight in the foods that He has created. Now that you are eating less often and less food, you will discover that eating primarily pleasers is a wonderful experience.

List some of your pleasers in the space below. Remember they are very specific.

_____

_____

_____

_____

The second category of food is called "teasers." In the average home the most readily available foods are teasers. Teasers are often what we grab when we are on the run and just want something—anything—to eat.

Teasers

1. They are convenient and easy to get.
2. They tend to call out and tempt you.
3. They are generally eaten when our flesh machinery is in high gear.
4. They look better than they taste.
5. They are not much more than a "stuffer" or a "filler," and we often overeat teasers for precisely that reason.
6. They are not very satisfying, making us think "more is better."
7. It is a food that wasn't on your mind until you heard about it, saw it, or smelled it.
8. The all-time classic teaser is what's left of your pleaser when you have reached your comfortable 5 and are satisfied!

There is another important difference between pleasers and teasers. When you wait until your body is truly hungry, it sends you clear messages as to what food you want to eat. This will usually be something you really enjoy (a true pleaser), and you will tend to eat just enough because it is so satisfying.

On the other hand, if you eat when you're not truly hungry (what we call "grazing"), you won't get a clear message from your body. You'll be inclined to go after teasers and will end up being totally unsatisfied. Our impulse is to eat more in order to try to experience satisfaction. Of course, the obvious solution is to wait until you are hungry and then to enjoy the appropriate pleasers.

Having said all of that, we are not telling you never to eat another teaser. As we've pointed out, all foods are permissible, even though some are not very beneficial. Just know that satisfaction is rarely found in eating teasers. With that in mind, you are better equipped to make more discerning food choices. You can establish food boundaries for yourself based on how the Lord leads you personally, moment-by-moment.

List some of your teasers in the space below.

_____

_____

The third category is called "total rejects." Some foods are simply not worth eating. They are too sweet, too salty, too fatty, artificially flavored, artificially colored, boring, unimaginative, don't-even-taste-good-yucky-foods with no redeeming qualities. There's no need to spend time talking about this one. Don't waste your 0, your time, or your money on them. They really are total rejects.

Total Rejects

List some total rejects you have eliminated over the last fourteen days.

Now we are ready to look at the bigger picture, which requires more discernment.

Whole-Body Pleasers

As you learn to listen to the signals from your God-given body, you may notice that many of your pleasers are nothing more than "taste-bud pleasers." Since you are more than taste buds, your body will have a desire for something we call a "whole-body pleaser." These are the foods that make you feel good overall. For instance, you may consider a hot fudge sundae one of your most pleasurable pleasers. However, if after you have eaten a hot fudge sundae you feel quite lethargic, then the sundae isn't a whole-body pleaser.

Another example would be strawberries. If you love the taste of fresh strawberries, but get a rash after you eat them, they are not a whole body pleaser for you. Or, suppose it's mid-morning and the smell of donuts fills the office. You are at a 0 so you eat a couple of them. But if after eating them you get a headache, then it's safe to say that donuts are not your whole body pleasers.

Whole-body pleasers are those foods that your body calls out for, are enjoyable while you eat them, and they leave you feeling energized afterward. As you become more sensitive to the signals your body sends you, your pleaser/teaser discernment will improve day by day.

Take Action

+ Deal wisely with teasers because they can complicate and interfere with conscious eating. Make room for pleasers that bring total satisfaction.
+ Don't fall back on teasers when you get into a "munchy" mode. If they aren't easily accessible, you won't be tempted. Eat only the choice foods that you enjoy.
+ Totally reject total rejects.

In the house of the wise are stores of choice food and oil, but a foolish man devours all he has (Proverbs 21:20).

It's amazing how different our lives become when we choose whole-body pleasers rather than fare that is second best. Elanya, a Thin Within participant tells us, "I used to try to lose weight by eating only salads without dressing, dry toast, hard boiled eggs, cooked cabbage, and boiled skinless chicken."

Do all of these sound like pleasers? We doubt it! Can you see more clearly why diets don't work? They are made up almost entirely of teasers and rejects. Rebecca on the other hand said she became more adventuresome with Thin Within and found out she liked eating flaxseed in her hot cereal and soybeans in her salads. New options opened up for her with the wisdom to make some creative choices.

The categories that we are establishing help define the boundary lines that have fallen in pleasant places for our bodies, the temple of God. We can refer to these categories in order to select those foods that are the most satisfying.

We must remain even more vigilant, however, regarding what satisfies our souls, which is intimacy with the Lord. Whole-body pleasers, regardless of the quantity, will never satisfy the emptiness that God wants to fill with His presence, power, and love. Let's continue to participate in this journey, which is strengthening and building your spirit, mind, and body as a temple for His glory.

My soul will be satisfied as with the richest of foods; with singing lips my mouth will praise you (Psalm 63:5).

Your Success Story

Did you have any new insights while you were reading today? Please record them below.

_____

_____

_____

Verses to Ponder

Let us discern for ourselves what is right; let us learn together what is good (Job 34:4).

The discerning heart seeks knowledge, but the mouth of a fool feeds on folly (Proverbs 15:14).

My son, preserve sound judgment and discernment, do not let them out of your sight (Proverbs 3:21).

Discretion will protect you, and understanding will guard you (Proverbs 2:11).

Prayer

Dear Lord, I'm so thankful that You want me to delight in the good foods that You have created. I pray, Lord, that I will respond to the signals sent to me by my body and that I won't allow a dieting mentality to keep me from a food that would be a whole-body pleaser. Lord, please give me strength and discernment where food choices are concerned, and please lead me by the power of Your Holy Spirit so that you can fill the emptiness in my soul with what would be pleasing to You. In Jesus' name, Amen.

Success Tools

+ Rate your foods as either pleasers or teasers in your food log. You can rate them from 0 (awful or total rejects) to 10 (fabulous).
+ Continue using your Observations and Corrections Chart.
+ Use the Thin Within Keys to Conscious Eating when you choose to eat or drink today.
+ Use the Hunger Graph to keep track of your eating today.

Medical Moment

The boundaries between science and faith are not nearly so clearly delineated as in the past. In ancient times and in primitive cultures, healing traditionally was in the hands of the priest or medicine man, whose "healing" involved invoking whichever god or gods were deemed appropriate. This practice continued pretty much unchallenged until modern times. Then science emerged and was widely accepted as holding the solution to the ills of humankind. This was especially true in the past one hundred years with so many advances by the scientific community. In recent years, however, there has been renewed interest in what might be called nontraditional healing, including the roles of spirituality and faith. There is now an ever-increasing body of medical literature documenting the role that our beliefs play in health, healing, and wellness, and an increasing number of medical schools are addressing this issue. It is a difficult area to examine using traditional scientific methods, but we firmly believe that faith and prayer are very important to our emotional and physical well-being and that more and more this will be acknowledged, documented and accepted in time.

—Arthur W. Halliday, M.D.

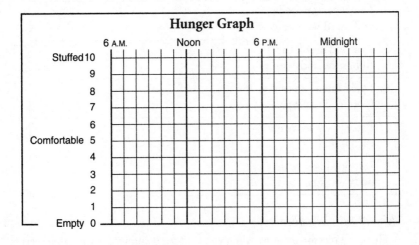

Thin Within Food Log

Hunger # before Eating	Time	Items/ Amount	Rate: Total Rejects (0) Pleasers (10)	Hunger # after Eating

Thin Within Observations and Corrections Chart—Day 18

Observations	Day 18
1. I ate when my body was hungry.	
2. I ate in a calm environment by reducing distractions.	
3. I ate when I was sitting.	
4. I ate when my body and mind were relaxed.	
5. I ate and drank the things my body enjoyed.	
6. I paid attention to my food while eating.	
7. I ate slowly, savoring each bite.	
8. I stopped before my body was full.	

Thin Within Wisdom

There is a blessing in store when you wait for 0 and feed it with a pleaser!

Opening the Prison Gates

Say to the captives, "Come out," and to those in darkness, "Be free!"
They will feed beside the roads and find pasture on every barren hill.
They will neither hunger nor thirst,
nor will the desert heat or the sun beat upon them.
He who has compassion on them will
guide them and lead them beside springs of water.
I will turn all my mountains into roads, and my highways will be raised up.
—Isaiah 49:9–11

We have laid a foundation and our restoration project is well underway with Christ as the cornerstone. The infrastructure is reinforced, the outer walls are complete. Now we move our attention to the inner walls. Here we will continue to build as we retain an attitude of vulnerability and humility, ever mindful that He is the master and we are the apprentices who serve at His side.

Jesus takes our hands in His and shows us how to chisel away each stone to ensure its proper fit. We feel His rough palms on our hands and we are reminded that our relationship with Him came at an incredible price. Nail scars on those calloused hands bear testimony that Jesus purchased our pardon when He willingly stretched out His arms on the cross in submission to His Father's will. He made it possible for us to forever enjoy the presence of God. Now He labors beside us in our restoration process.

In His presence, pause and consider Isaiah's encounter with God, when he saw the Lord in Heavenly splendor and majesty. Isaiah's response to this vision was *Woe to me! . . . I am ruined! For I am a man of unclean lips, and I live among a people of unclean lips, and my eyes have seen the King, the* LORD *Almighty* (Isaiah 6:5).

It is inevitable that we should experience humility and vulnerability in the presence of God. Simon Peter fished all night without so much as a nibble. Jesus told him to put out his nets again. Peter obeyed and the nets began to break due to the unbelievable catch of fish that followed. Knowing that he stood not before a man, but before God, Peter responded in the only way possible. He fell at Jesus' feet and said, *Go away from me, Lord; I am a sinful man!* (Luke 5:8)

In Jesus' presence we become keenly aware of our own shortcomings and sin, yet this awareness is immediately overshadowed by affirmation and loving-kindness of a gracious God.

"Your guilt is taken away and your sin atoned for." Then I heard the voice of the Lord saying, "Whom shall I send? And who will go for us?" And I said, "Here am I. Send me!" He said, "Go . . ." (Isaiah 6:7b–9a).

God sends or commissions us when we have an understanding of Him as master and ourselves as apprentices and when we recognize all that He has so generously given.

What is the single greatest gift that God has bestowed on humankind? There can be no doubt that it is the forgiveness of all our sins in Christ. John MacArthur, Jr., says it well: "There would be no salvation, relationship to God, entering into heaven, no usefulness to God, and no relief of guilt, without the forgiveness of sin."[1]

Further, there would be no indwelling presence, no experience of His comfort and peace without the forgiveness of sin. We would be shattered by the awareness of our own sin without the revelation that we are now complete in Christ. *Praise be to the God and Father of our Lord Jesus Christ* (2 Corinthians 1:3a).

Our God has provided a way for us to have an accurate assessment of ourselves without being undone in the process. This is the very reason that He provided the Lamb of God to take away the sins of the world. It was *while* we were yet sinners that Christ died for the ungodly (Romans 5:8).

In repentance and rest is your salvation, in quietness and trust is your strength (Isaiah 30:15).

When we acknowledge that we have chosen to do what is right in our own eyes, such as eat that third donut, we have made a choice in the flesh. We stand in agreement with God and confess that we have made a detour from the path of God's provision. If our hearts are open to Him, we will see that the scenery is much grander back on His path. So we humbly admit to Him that we have wandered off the road.

This is the first step of repentance.

The second step is taken when we turn our backs away from our sin and turn, instead, toward God, realigning ourselves to His purposes and His will.

Repentance means, if you get on the path of your performance, you intentionally turn back to Him and onto the path of His provision. And it is in this process of observation (which is confession) and correction (which is repentance) that you find His strength in the place of your weakness. Even your willingness to acknowledge your sin and turn to God is a work that He performs in you (Acts 5:31; Acts 11:18).

Those who oppose him he must gently instruct, in the hope that God will grant them repentance leading them to a knowledge of the truth (2 Timothy 2:25).

It is God's loving-kindness that leads us to repentance. We will be welcomed with mercy, grace, and tenderness when we run into His arms. God's kindness leads us to turn back and stand in agreement with Him, "Yes, this is sin." We then are able to say, "Lord, I repent. I return to you because I long to do what You desire for me."

In this place our sins, none of which are beyond the reach of His grace, are wiped away and we are blessedly and totally refreshed in His commands (Acts 3:19).

Blessed is he whose transgressions are forgiven, whose sins are covered. Blessed is the man whose sin the LORD does not count against him and in whose spirit is no deceit (Psalm 32:1–2).

In light of so great a salvation, how then shall we respond to our own sin? God paid an enormous price for our freedom, yet we sometimes have difficulty accepting His gift. We may think that the blood of Christ will cover everyone's sins but our own. Or we may believe in the theory of God's forgiveness, but in practice, we are unable to receive it in our own hearts.

Do you realize that nothing can separate you from the love of Christ (Romans 8:35, 38, 39)? God doesn't look upon our sin with approval, but He does look upon it with a solution. He disapproves of our sin but *not of us*. The one who mandates that we forgive up to "seventy times seven" (Matthew 18:22), forgives our every offense.

Louise, a Thin Within participant who released over fifty pounds, shares, "How freeing it was finally to understand that if I am willing and sincere in taking that first step, the Lord holds my hand during the entire journey and that nothing can separate me from His love. Nothing I have done is so horrible that He won't forgive me and welcome me back into His loving arms."

The woman at the well met the Lord at midday because her shame kept her from going out in public when the other women drew water. Once she had met Him, she declared to the others, *Come and see a man who told me everything I ever did. Could this be the Christ?* (John 4:29). Jesus knew all about the woman, and yet He met her with such gentleness and love that she longed for others to meet Him as well.

In an account of another woman who struggled with sin, we see a different example of Jesus' grace. Cynthia Heald tells the story in a unique way:

> Jesus, full of grace and truth, was in the temple. The Jewish legalists, seeking to trap Him, brought to Him a woman caught in the act of adultery. The Law spoke to Grace: "She has broken the law. The law says she should die. What do you say?"
>
> Grace replied to the Law, "If you have not sinned, you can stone her."
>
> And because the law reveals sin, those who were under it were exposed, and they left.
>
> Grace turned to the sinner and asked, "Where are your accusers? Is there no one who condemns you?" The sinner, in the presence of Grace, saw that she was no longer accused. Then she heard the pronouncement of freedom and forgiveness: "Neither do I. Go and sin no more."[2]

The Lord knows all about us. He doesn't want us to hang on to the shame, pain, and wounds of our past. Nor does He want us to deny our sin and remain distant from Him. Instead He longs for us to come before His throne of grace to receive mercy and find grace to help us in our time of need (Hebrews 4:16).

Debra writes, "At Thin Within I looked at what was causing me to eat more than my body needed, and I saw that going to food for comfort was a coping mechanism. So now instead of overeating, I go to God and tell Him I should have come to Him in the first place. He is always there, ready to forgive me. I want to receive His forgiveness instead of getting stuck in the cycle of, 'Since I have already eaten too much, I may as well eat more.'"

Resting and trusting in the Lord's forgiveness is an invaluable aspect of His restoration work within us. He wants to lift you up no matter how many times you stumble. He speaks gently, "I don't condemn you. Leave your life of sin." He beckons you to walk with Him, to speak openly with Him about your struggles and about your shame. He wants to lift your countenance and raise your vision until all you can see is His face, full of love for you.

Shake off your dust; rise up, sit enthroned, O Jerusalem. Free yourself from the chains on your neck, O captive Daughter of Zion (Isaiah 52:2).

Your Savior beckons you to draw near to Him with confidence. He calls to you to shake off the dust, rise up as His beloved child, and sit enthroned. You have been held captive, perhaps, but in this moment, God has ordained from eternity past that you would be still before Him and choose to receive fully the blessings of His forgiveness. Will you step forward out of the shackles? Will you choose to believe what He has said in His Word about you? He enfolds you with His love. He forgives your every sin. He washes away all impurity.

Let's apply these truths to our lives in this very moment. Don't miss this opportunity to draw nearer to the heart of God.

Take Action

+ For the past eighteen days you have had the freedom to use or not to use the observation and correction charts, food logs, hunger graphs, and records of your flesh machinery. You have traveled far, so let's look back over your Thin Within journey. Note any way in which you feel disappointment with yourself. Is there anything over the past eighteen days for which you need to forgive yourself?

+ Rather than pulling out the "club of condemnation" pull out the "tool" of forgiveness provided for you by the cross of Christ. Use the lines below to make a list of things for which you will forgive yourself.

_____

_____

_____

+ Pray about these things and ask God to remove any self-condemnation or shame. Thank Him that He has already done so.

+ Turn now to the Significant Times Exercise in Day Sixteen and prayerfully consider the role you have played in your food, eating, or weight problems. List everything that comes to your mind, including things where you experienced shame even in situations where you may not have been primarily at fault.

The purpose of this exercise is to identify any sins (perceived or legitimate) for which you have been punishing yourself. The enemy stands in accusation, but Jesus is your defense attorney. Remember the Lord already knows about all our transgressions and has paid the penalty for them. On the cross He carried not only our sin, but also our shame. If you don't feel comfortable writing this in your book, use a separate sheet of paper and burn it after you are finished.

I Choose to Receive God's Forgiveness for Myself for

_____

_____

_____

_____

_____

_____

If we confess our sins, he is faithful and just to forgive us our sins, and to cleanse us from all unrighteousness (1 John 1:9, KJV).

+ Pray, as you bring each of the items you listed to the Lord. He wants to lighten your burden, which isn't yours alone to carry. He carries it with you.
+ Receive the forgiveness that has been freely given to you.
+ Write forgiveness phrases for yourself for each of the things you identified above. For example: "In obedience to God, I, (your name), choose to forgive myself as Christ forgives me for using food as my refuge rather than running to God."

_____

_____

_____

_____

_____

_____

_____

_____

_____

_____

_____

✦ What insights did you have from this exercise?

_____

_____

_____

_____

Now is the time to release whatever may be standing in your way of receiving God's total and complete forgiveness established for you at the Cross. You are *not* an exception. God has the power to cleanse you whiter than snow. Jesus' blood covers all your sin, and He points you toward the future with new resolve and power to become all that He calls you to be.

For the grace of God that brings salvation has appeared to all men. It teaches us to say "No" to ungodliness and worldly passions, and to live self-controlled, upright and godly lives in this present age, while we wait for the blessed hope— the glorious appearing of our great God and Savior, Jesus Christ, who gave himself for us to redeem us from all wickedness and to purify for himself a people that are his very own, eager to do what is good (Titus 2:11–14).

In this place of total cleansing, as in Isaiah 6, we hear the commissioning of our God: "Who will go?" We have the blessed opportunity to respond: "Send me."

As we step forward in faith, we answer His call to holiness. We are asked by Jesus to "go and leave this life of sin." As we step forward in faith, leaving behind that which entangled us, grace enfolds us. As we run with perseverance the race marked out for us, grace embraces us. As we fix our eyes on the author and perfector of our faith, grace envelops us. As we set our sights on things above, not on earthly things, grace continually abounds around us. Grace covers all of our sin and gives us all we need to press on, fulfilling His plan and purpose.

Your Success Story

Did you have any new insights while you were reading today? Please record them below.

_____

_____

_____

Verses to Ponder

Blessed is he whose transgressions are forgiven, whose sins are covered. Blessed is the man whose sin the LORD does not count against him and in whose spirit is no deceit. When I kept silent, my bones wasted away through my groaning all day long. For day and night your hand was heavy upon me; my strength was sapped as in the heat of summer. Then I acknowledged my sin to you and did not cover up my iniquity. I said, "I will confess my transgressions to the LORD"—and you forgave the guilt of my sin (Psalm 32:1–5).

The Spirit of the Sovereign LORD is on me, because the LORD has anointed me to preach good news to the poor. He has sent me to bind up the broken-hearted, to proclaim freedom for the captives and release from darkness for the prisoners (Isaiah 61:1).

The LORD hears the needy and does not despise his captive people (Psalm 69:33).

Prayer

Oh, Lord, thank You so much for giving Yourself specifically for me so that I am completely forgiven. Thank You for Your amazing grace that extends from Your throne as a powerful covering affecting all I do. I pray that I will not think that my sin is beyond the scope and expanse of Your mercy and forgiveness. I pray that I will not harbor resentment toward myself that can turn into self-pity or into anger toward You. Help me to release any unforgiving feelings toward myself, feelings that would imply that the blood You shed on the cross at Calvary wasn't enough to cover my sins. Thank You, Lord, that You paid it all. In Jesus' name, Amen.

Medical Moment

In spite of the vast distribution of information about what constitutes a healthy lifestyle and despite medical advances being realized in certain areas, the overall health of Americans can be greatly improved. The focus of our ministry is on total body health—physical, emotional, and spiritual, based on the biblical mandate that we are to be good stewards of all of God's creation, including ourselves. Christ said, "Whatever you do to the least of my brethren, that you do to me" (Matthew 25:40). And the famous psychiatrist, Carl Jung asked the penetrating question, "What if this least of brethren is you?" Think about it—what we do to ourselves we do also to Him, Christ in us. Some of the ills of humankind are the result of things beyond our control—genetic abnormalities, accidents, etc., but we have direct control of many areas of our health. Sadly it is estimated that hundreds of thousands of lives are lost in this country each year because of improper (usually "over") eating, inadequate exercise, and substance abuse. Fortunately much of this is avoidable when we treat our body with the honor and respect to which we are commissioned by God.

—ARTHUR HALLIDAY, M.D.

Success Tools

+ Feel free to continue using the Hunger Graph.
+ Fill in the Thin Within Food Log.
+ Mark the Thin Within Observations and Corrections Chart for today.
+ Use the Thin Within Keys to Conscious Eating when you choose to eat or drink today.

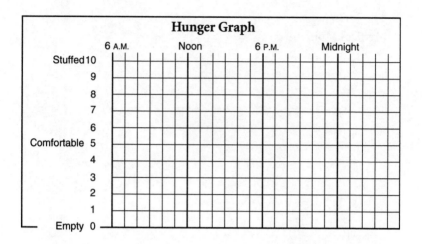

Thin Within Food Log

Hunger # before Eating	Time	Items/Amount	Hunger # after Eating

Thin Within Observations and Corrections Chart—Day 19

Observations	Day 19
1. I ate when my body was hungry.	
2. I ate in a calm environment by reducing distractions.	
3. I ate when I was sitting.	
4. I ate when my body and mind were relaxed.	
5. I ate and drank the things my body enjoyed.	
6. I paid attention to my food while eating.	
7. I ate slowly, savoring each bite.	
8. I stopped before my body was full.	

Thin Within Wisdom

Grace teaches us to say "no" to ungodly choices.

God's kindness leads us toward repentance.

NOTES

1. John MacArthur, Jr., *The Restoration of a Sinning Saint*, n.p., n.d.
2. Cynthia Heald, *Becoming a Woman of Grace* (Nashville, Tennessee: Thomas Nelson Publishers, 1998), 46.

Release of the Captives

*Bear with each other
and forgive whatever grievances you may have against one another.
Forgive as the Lord forgave you.*
—Colossians 3:13

We are thrilled to have walked side by side with you these past nineteen days. Our prayer is that you are seeing the glory of God's restoration reflected in your body as His magnificent temple. Now we will deal the enemy a harsh blow. This is an exciting day that breathes of hope beyond measure. As with anything worth obtaining, we may find ourselves up to our elbows in desert dust, but there is a stream of pure water, flowing from the throne of our God, that cleanses and purifies us.

Let us take stock of all that has been accomplished in the strength of the Lord during the past nineteen days. We have chosen to stand on God's truth, the foundation He has laid. We believe that what God says is true. We know we can appropriate His gifts of grace, mercy, and forgiveness and be loosed from the shackles of shame and guilt. Jesus has declared us "not guilty." He has called us to be holy as He is holy (1 Peter 1:15–16). As we walk in the confidence that God is right and what He says is true, we know that we can do all things through Christ who strengthens us (Philippians 4:13).

But there is one last caution that needs to be stated so that we can fully experience our freedom. Look again at the analogy of the eagle and imagine our eagle reflecting on his previous life as a chicken. He thinks, "Now wait just a minute, I *thought* I was a chicken all those years because Aunt Tillie always told me so. Dad convinced me that I needed to scratch for my food, and my sister Sylvia persuaded me that life was meant to be lived in a chicken coop." Suddenly our eagle has become aware that many of the beliefs that shaped his actions and the subsequent results came from others in his life.

What's an eagle to do when he realizes that some of the beliefs that shaped his life came about as a result of sin (intentional or unintentional) of those around him? As our eagle analogy ends, we are faced with a ponderous question. Do we let the pronouncements of others keep us locked in a "chicken" mentality? Or do we let God use those very things to strengthen us so that we might spread our wings to their full expanse and fly. We must prevent bitterness from taking root in our hearts and receive the fullness of God's grace and extend forgiveness to those who have wronged us (Hebrews 12:15). If we are to walk in lifelong freedom on the path of God's provision, we will soon see that it is also a path of forgiveness.

"My father always acted as if I were in his way and he never had time for me. I had little nurturing from an emotionally unstable mother and believed I was worthless. As a child, I felt that if I could just be good enough, all the problems in my family would go away. I felt like it was my fault—that I was ruining everyone's lives," confides Lucia, who had long battled with her weight and a very low self-image when she came to Thin Within.

Lucia continues, "When I chose deliberately to forgive my parents, I spent time journaling each and every offense that I held against them, and I prayerfully released each offense to the Lord. Jesus paid with his blood for their sins, just as He did for mine. I was amazed at the freedom I then experienced in my eating as a result. Suddenly food didn't have the hold that it had for so long. I really don't fully understand it, but I know what happened was miraculous. After months of trying so hard to deal with my issues with food and eating, when I forgave my dad and mom, suddenly I walked in freedom. As I released my parents, I released the excess weight."

Lucia discovered that there was a key that unlocked the fetters that had previously remained solidly in place. That key was forgiveness.

Yesterday we looked at the need to receive God's forgiveness and to commit ourselves to moving forward in the strength He provides. Today we shift the focus a bit to look upon Christ, our Savior, who died for the sins of the whole world.

Many times we don't want to acknowledge that others have wounded us, thinking that it isn't "biblical" to feel hurt, much less to express that hurt. However, as we observed on Day Eighteen, having godly boundaries doesn't mean putting our heads in the sand but rather protecting that which God has entrusted to us. When we are wounded and choose to deal with the pain and speak about it, we are acknowledging an appropriate biblical boundary. In Christ, we can admit the truth instead of pretending that something traumatic didn't happen, or that it didn't bother us.

It is important for us to avoid a sort of "sanctified denial" about the hurts of our past. This occurs when we generically tell God that we forgive _____ for being "so awful" or for being "abusive" without genuinely dealing with the truth about the person's actions or the subsequent wounds. If we refuse to face the facts, we will remain stuck in painful past events and the emotions attached to those events.

For instance, Lucia noted, "I wondered why I continued to have run-ins with women at church and at work. I discovered that, until I dealt with my anger toward my mother, I would have trouble responding to women in authority. I was treating them as if they had the characteristics of my mother—as if they were my mother."

Once Lucia dealt with the source of her feelings, she stopped reliving the situations in which her mother, her original authority figure, had abandoned her emotionally. She says, "I began to see each woman as an individual, and I was freed from treating them with the same resentment I had felt for my mom. Given that I always ate over these sorts of clashes, it is now clear to me why I began to eat much less once I had forgiven her."

Consider for a moment a cardiac patient facing heart transplant surgery. Certainly there is fear and concern. However, in her current circumstances she knows she will never again be able to enjoy running road races with her husband, downhill skiing with her kids, or mountain biking with her best friends. If she is willing to submit to the scalpel of a very talented heart surgeon, she will suffer discomfort and pain, but the end result will be a life of freedom and enjoyment for which she longs.

We, too, have an opportunity to lie upon the operating table. The Great Physician will probe and open our hearts. He will shine His light in those dark corners of our hearts. In fact, Scripture says He will perform a heart transplant, giving us a new heart, removing our heart of stone (Ezekiel 11:19). Can you imagine? After a heart transplant like that, we would be "good to go" for this amazing adventure called the abundant life.

Carla released forty pounds during her experience with Thin Within. As to the importance of forgiveness in her healing process, Carla said, "I learned how to forgive my mother for always having me on a diet, and I accepted the fact that she had done the best she could, considering her own background. She had a weight problem in college and managed to lose weight, but she didn't want a fat daughter. So I grew up with a lot of anger from the age of eleven or twelve."

As you face the reasons you turn to food, you can turn to God for His wisdom and healing. You can trust Him to nurture and restore you to full spiritual, emotional, and physical health.

Peter tells of his own need to forgive, "When I was only ten, a boy just a few years older than I molested me repeatedly. Twenty-five years later, when I realized how this affected me, the first step toward my recovery was to forgive the molester. It was painful but necessary."

People like Peter and Carla had to make a conscious decision. They chose to look at their lives during childhood and adolescence, not to dig up dirt, but in an honest, godly attempt to understand what had happened that prompted them to feel anger and rebellion and to abuse food, eating, and their bodies. As they did, they realized that they had, in effect, been held captive by those who had wronged them. When they forgave those involved, they were released from many of the issues that triggered unconscious eating. In effect, as the heart transplant took hold, they obtained a softened heart toward those who had wronged them and in the process were given a new life of joy and freedom.

Earlier, when we looked at our flesh machinery, we discovered that many factors play a role in who we are today. Out of our past stories have emerged beliefs that powerfully affect our actions. Ultimately this determines what we believe about ourselves. When carefully considered, the past can have a tremendous impact on how we relate to food and our bodies.

Claudia recalls, "My mom taught us some bad eating habits. She grazed all the time and ate constantly while cooking. She also ate all the leftovers after dinner. The forgiveness exercises at Thin Within helped me forgive her for being overweight herself and for passing that legacy on to me."

Claudia's upbringing affected the way she viewed meal preparation and food in general. She felt resentment toward her mother for her own weight problem. However, as she realized this and took steps to forgive her mother, she walked in freedom and released over forty pounds.

Let's call a purposeful halt to allowing the wounds of the past to affect our eating today. In fact, we want to stop what happened fifteen years ago, an hour ago, or fifteen minutes ago, from determining how we respond to food in the present moment.

Yesterday we looked at the fact that Jesus extends forgiveness to each of us. We hope and pray that you chose to receive for yourself the grace and forgiveness that flows freely from the cross of Christ.

In today's exercise, we will extend forgiveness to others. We will sever those remaining links of the chain that have bound you to the past. First, however, let's examine what forgiveness actually is and what it is not.

What Forgiveness Is and Is Not

1. Forgiveness is *not* letting the wrongdoer off the hook. "Once I forgave my husband for his infidelity, I came to realize that one day he will stand before God, knowing his guilt completely," shares Julia. "Rather than 'letting him off,' I realized I only released Him into God's hands." God is our judge and as we entrust ourselves to Him who judges justly, He will apportion the correct justice to those around us (1 Peter 2:23).

2. Forgiveness *does* release the right to get revenge. If we are honest, much of our lack of forgiveness comes from desiring to take things in our own hands and get the revenge that we think is justified. However, the Bible reminds us that God canceled our debt against Him and that if we got what we deserved, it would be death (Romans 6:23; Colossians 2:13–14). It only stands to reason that we would be called to release those for whom Christ purchased a pardon.

Do not repay anyone evil for evil. . . . Do not take revenge, my friends, but leave room for God's wrath, for it is written: "It is mine to avenge; I will repay" (Romans 12:17a, 19).

3. Forgiveness is *not* forgetting. Many people feel that if you don't forget you haven't forgiven. This isn't necessarily the case. God may erase it from your mind. However, on the other hand, it may not be beneficial for you to forget, so God may *not* erase it from your memory.

Diane had struggled for years with anorectic and bulimic behavior. She explains, "I had no memory of being sexually abused as a child, but I had all the symptoms. My counselor told me that he suspected that I had been molested, but that just made me angry. One night, when a physician I was dating kissed me, I had a flashback. He told me that he had seen the behavior I exhibited in patients who had been molested. I went to a post-traumatic stress disorder clinic for adults molested as children. There I realized that it wasn't only the memories that were missing. What was also missing was the realization that what had happened to me was *not* 'normal.'"

As Diane came to terms with the truth about the abuse, she was able to walk in the freedom of forgiveness. God restored her memory in His perfect timing as she was able to cope with it, so that His purposes could be accomplished in her. We are called to forgive but not always to forget. God, however, is the one who forgives and forgets.

I, even I, am he who blots out your transgressions, for my own sake, and remembers your sins no more (Isaiah 43:25).

The Lord doesn't store up a record of our wrongs so that at just the opportune moment He can lower the boom. He simply forgives us. To be Christlike, we also are called to pursue forgiveness.

If you, O LORD, kept a record of sins, O Lord, who could stand? But with you there is forgiveness (Psalm 130:3–4a).

4. Forgiveness is *not* a feeling. It is an act of obedience that we offer to the Lord. Feelings, however, may eventually follow as we step out in faith. In order to avoid turning forgiveness into "sanctified denial," as we mentioned earlier, we must acknowledge our pain, giving it a voice and inviting the Lord to bind up our broken hearts.

We humble ourselves in the sight of God and trust Him to lift us up. With every suffering that surfaces, we come to the Lord, palms open, heart broken, asking him to show us how we are to respond. What personal characteristics has that wound shaped? What coping mechanisms did you develop to protect yourself when, perhaps, you knew no alternative?

Search me, O God, and know my heart; test me and know my anxious thoughts. See if there is any offensive way in me, and lead me in the way everlasting (Psalm 139:23–24).

As we offer our wounded hearts to God, He shows us how insults or wounds to our souls and spirits as children, adolescents, adults—even in yesterday's interaction at the post office or on the freeway—may have left us with a bitter residue. Pain can penetrate deeply into who we are, affecting our beliefs, our actions, and the subsequent results. Some of us have responded by trying in our own strength to cope and endure the pain as best we can. However, in doing so, we may have turned to behaviors that are inappropriate or destructive, or that have become strongholds of sin.

What is a stronghold? "Strongholds keep us from being free to reflect Christ in and through our lives because they require allegiance until they are dealt with. Strongholds can often be so hidden that we would not even identify them as evil. A stronghold of fear, control, rebellion, insecurity, idolatry, pride, or bitterness may be hidden until it is revealed through circumstances. All strongholds are built in our lives as a result of seeking to meet one or more of the basic needs God has created in us. Once we believe a lie that God cannot meet a need without our effort, we open our spirit to a stronghold. The more lies we believe, the more we invite these strongholds to take root in our lives."

An example can be found in the "rager," someone in whom rage has a "strong hold." A rager gets angry and lashes out at anyone close at hand when he feels a lack of control. His rage often covers a great deal of pain. By lashing out he attempts to deflect his own pain and to numb himself to the wound in his soul. In this way, he seeks to control others, which gives him a sense of power.

As a child, rage may have helped him survive. As an adult, however, it won't work. At any point, the one who rages may choose to invite the Spirit of the Lord to enlighten his mind and receive the help needed to honestly deal with his emotions so he can leave this destructive behavior behind.

Another example of a stronghold of sin is compulsive overeating. Many tend to view overeating as socially acceptable, however God's Word has rightly warned against "greed" and "gluttony" because of the physical, emotional, and spiritual consequences of such choices. *But among you there must not be even a hint of sexual immorality, or any kind of impurity, or of greed, because these are improper for God's holy people* (Ephesians 5:3). Proverbs 23:21 reminds us that *drunkards and gluttons become poor, and drowsiness clothes them in rags.* Many tend to use food as an anesthetic, an escape, or a source of comfort much like alcohol or drugs or excessive work. If you know in your heart you turn to food instead of to God to meet your needs, then overeating may be a stronghold in your life. If we face those things that we may be avoiding or that cause us pain, and if we forgive others and ourselves, we are less likely to resort to abusing food and our bodies.

In order to forgive others, we must walk through the pain, seeking to acknowledge how it has affected and hurt us and how we have responded to it in present time. With our hand in God's hand, He will lead us through this valley of the shadow to the other side where we can be free to experience present time eating and where we will dwell in the house of the Lord forever (Psalm 23).[1]

5. Forgiveness *does* embrace the offender.

Jesus said, "Father, forgive them, for they do not know what they are doing" (Luke 23:34).

Forgiveness gives up control and is willing to release the offense into God's hands. This requires vulnerability and humility. If you struggle to forgive, the Lord knows and understands. The solution is to pray, asking Him to help you be willing to be made willing.

6. Forgiveness *is* making a choice. There is one crucial step to the process of forgiving: Trust God!

With the knowledge that it is what God has called us to do, even though we may not feel like it, fully understand it, or want to do it, we do it anyway out of love, obedience, and trust in our sovereign God.

Bear with each other and forgive whatever grievances you may have against one another. Forgive as the Lord forgave you (Colossians 3:13).

The price Jesus paid for our forgiveness motivates us to extend forgiveness to others as well. If not, I am, essentially, declaring His sacrifice insufficient to pay for the wrong done against me. His heart aches as He wants us to be freed from the pain and anger our souls have suffered at the hands of others. He wants us to experience true freedom (Galatians 5:1).

7. Forgiveness is something I choose to do. It is done deliberately as an obedient act of the will. It doesn't wait for the offender to initiate or behave in a certain way. This is especially crucial for those living with the very ones who have wronged them.

Sometimes we are able to forgive the past, but we find ourselves challenged when the hurtful person continues to wound us. We wonder, "I have forgiven them, now why can't they change?" As understandable as this may seem, God in His sovereignty has another plan. He may allow this difficult person to be His tool to refine us. As we continue in trust, forgiving in each present moment, keeping no record of wrongs, God will be faithful and just to work His good through our situation.

We certainly are not advocating that anyone remain in an abusive situation. However, even there, forgiveness can be extended, knowing the consequences for the abuse are in the hands of a just God. It is necessary, in order to keep yourself and your loved ones safe and to encourage healing for the abuser, to establish and maintain appropriate boundaries.

Linda recalls, "I chose to forgive my husband for his sexual addiction. However, I also laid out some clear boundaries. For him to remain in the household, which is what we both wanted, he had to pursue an active plan of recovery. I wouldn't have him endangering our children through a temptation of molestation, or me through the risk of HIV. He had to commit to and remain involved with active recovery if he were to remain in our home. If not, he would have to leave until he did. Many friends thought this was an ungodly boundary. I felt, however, that this was God's plan for us—to remain together but seek healing. Too many things are possible when sex addiction isn't brought under the healing power of the Spirit. I am blessed to say, three years later, he has been set free and our marriage is stronger than ever."

Linda's boundaries didn't imply that she wasn't willing to forgive; however, there were consequences that came as a result of her husband's behavior. It was, in fact, prayer and appropriate boundary setting that allowed both Linda and her husband to experience forgiveness and God's bountiful blessings in their surrendered obedience.

8. Forgiveness does *not* mean reconciliation (which requires participation of both parties). You don't necessarily need to be in an active relationship with the offender. In fact, the offender may no longer be alive. As we choose with an act of our will to release those who have wounded us something marvelous occurs. We discover that it is we who are released. In fact, the people who wronged us were never really held captive by our lack of forgiveness. It is we who were both the captor and the captive—locked up in a self-imposed prison of our own making.

As we choose to own the pain of another's sins against us, we experience freedom from resentment, bitterness, anger, and from the desire for revenge. Peace permeates our hearts where once there was discord. Many of the emotions that result in flesh machinery and inappropriate eating can be eliminated through the avenue of purposeful and prayerful forgiveness. As we respond to the Lord in trust and obedience, and as we offer Him our hearts and our wounds, He will bless our sincere desire to please Him.

Set me free from my prison, that I may praise your name. Then the righteous will gather about me because of your goodness to me (Psalm 142:7).

As we forgive, we will see Psalm 142:7 in action. We are released from our prison and our "chicken coop" mentality. We take to the sky and never look back. Our countenance is lighter and brighter. We are truly set free.

Take Action
+ My Forgiveness List

In Day Sixteen, you identified four "Significant Times" that affected you and your habits related to your body and food. With each situation, there was a list of people involved. In the space below, list the people in those four significant times against whom you harbor resentments. Invite God into this process, as He may lead you to include someone that you had not previously considered.

My Forgiveness List

_____

_____

_____

+ Write Forgiveness Phrases

Write forgiveness phrases for each of the people you identified. For example:

"I, (your name), out of obedience to God forgive _____, for the manipulation I experienced from critical and hurtful comments. I take back ground given to the enemy through my bitterness and yield that ground to the control of the Lord Jesus Christ."[2]

The more specific and detailed you can be the better. Continue to invite God into this process. Use the space provided, and blank sheets of paper if you need them. If you are not yet ready to forgive someone toward whom you know you harbor resentment, write a prayer asking that God make you willing to do so.

Write the forgiveness phrases many times (ten to twenty) daily until you experience release. I did this exercise over a period of approximately a year for hurtful things I experienced in my relationship with my father. It was amazing to me that suddenly one day I just knew it was finished. Our relationship was restored by the mercies of the Lord, which are new every morning.

_____

_____

_____

_____

_____

_____

✦ Let's move closer to the present moment now. Is there someone with whom you live or interact on a daily basis against whom you have been harboring unforgiveness? Remember that Jesus purchased both your freedom and his or hers. Write a prayer to God freeing the one who has wronged you. Will you release your anger, expectations, and unmet needs as you surrender them to your just and loving Heavenly Father?

_____

_____

_____

✦ What is your response to this exercise?

_____

_____

_____

It is our prayer that you will experience God's power as you forgive. It may seem impossible, but the faith that moves mountains can move your heart toward forgiveness; it will also move you toward a new view of food and your body. Ask for His help if you find yourself resisting.

"I had no clue that forgiving my brother was going to be the key that would unlock my bondage to compulsive overeating," states Christine, another Thin Within participant. "It wasn't until a summer of brokenness and crying out to the Lord to make the pain stop that I realized the answer to my 'What now, Lord?' question was 'Release him, my child.'

"As I wrote out forgiveness statements for each and every thing that I could think of that my brother had done to hurt me, I found myself still in tears, but the weight on my heart was beginning to lighten. I could then see, as never before, the connection between my eating and my upbringing. I was stuffing myself with food because of the pain of my childhood. I truly saw the Lord deliver me in those moments when I chose with my will to forgive. I thought I was freeing my brother, but I was really freeing myself from a self-imposed prison." Christine continues to walk in this place of freedom and she continues to release weight as well.

This journey is a training mission. We are being built stronger in the Lord much like a runner is built stronger through pushing just a bit farther than is comfortable. Going one more mile reaps great rewards. Pressing on through discomfort or even painful moments results in *strengthening* the physical body. If you have ever taken on a new exercise program or trained for a sporting event, you know what we mean. The actual muscle tissue of the body swells, resulting in muscle soreness sometimes twelve to thirty-six hours after the training session. The pain doesn't *feel* beneficial. However, what occurs is that the tiny muscle fibers causing the pain subsequently "hypertrophy," or enlarge, resulting in greater *strength*.

On our Thin Within journey we encourage you to press on through the discomfort. We don't want to minimize the pain you may be experiencing as you face the need to forgive others who have wronged you. However, we want to encourage you to see that there is so much more involved than what you see or feel in this moment. We find that in pressing on through the discomfort, the tearing down that you experience will actually result in a building up—a strengthening—of your body, soul, spirit, and mind. In short, your temple is becoming a more suitable dwelling place for the glory of the Lord Almighty.

Your Success Story

Did you have any new insights while you were reading today? Please record them below.

_____

_____

_____

Verses to Ponder

And when you stand praying, if you hold anything against anyone, forgive him, so that your Father in heaven may forgive you your sins (Mark 11:25).

In him we have redemption through his blood, the forgiveness of sins, in accordance with the riches of God's grace that he lavished on us with all wisdom and understanding (Ephesians 1:7–8).

Then Peter came to Jesus and asked, "Lord, how many times shall I forgive my brother when he sins against me? Up to seven times?" Jesus answered, "I tell you, not seven times, but seventy-seven times" (Matthew 18:21–22).

Prayer

O, Lord, make me willing always to forgive a wrong done to me. I want to be tenderhearted toward those who have offended me as well as those whom I've offended. This is so hard for me, Lord, because I admit at times I feel justified in my anger, resentment, and desire for revenge. Help me to trust You and know You will be fair and just. I know that as I step forward in faith to forgive, I will be free. That is my heart's desire. In Jesus' name I pray, Amen.

Success Tools

- ✦ Fill in the Hunger Graph.
- ✦ Fill in the Thin Within Food Log.
- ✦ Use the Thin Within Observations and Corrections Chart for today.
- ✦ Use the Thin Within Keys to Conscious Eating.

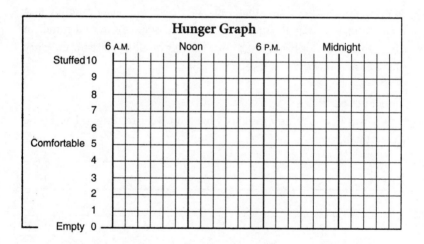

Hunger Graph

Thin Within **Wisdom**

Please don't underestimate the power of forgiveness.
It really *will* set you free.

Medical Moment

Fifty million Americans have hypertension and thirty million of them are at risk for heart attacks and strokes because their blood pressure is poorly controlled. Most hypertension is called "essential," which means that no specific cause can be found, but the prevailing belief is that the most common cause is chronic stress. There are many strategies recommended for stress relief, and each of us needs to appropriate whatever works best. In our experience, the relief of stress from forgiveness (of others and ourselves) is very effective.

Blood pressure is often labeled as follows for adults over eighteen years of age.

	Systolic Pressure	Diastolic Pressure
1. Optimal	<120	<80
2. Normal	<130	<85
3. High Normal	130–139	86–89
4. Milder Hypertension	140–159	90–99
5. Moderate Hypertension	160–179	100–109
6. Severe Hypertension	>180	>110

The things you can do to lower your blood pressure include:

1. Optimize your weight.

2. Stop smoking.

3. Get regular exercise several times a week.

4. Limit caffeine intake (coffee, chocolate, many soft drinks, many over-the-counter drugs—read the labels).

5. Avoid stress.

6. Get adequate sleep.

7. Avoid excessive salt intake.

Sometimes it is necessary to take anti-hypertensive medication.

It is important to have your blood pressure checked periodically and to cooperate fully with any prescribed treatment. Many **Thin Within** participants find that as they release their extra weight their blood pressure does return to the normal range.

—ARTHUR HALLIDAY, M.D.

NOTES

1. Os Hillman, *Today God is First—Marketplace Mediations* (Shippensburg, Pennsylvania: Destiny Image Publishers, 2000), 326.
2. Biblical Concept in Counseling, *People Who Have Hurt Me*, 2-A.

Thin Within Food Log

Hunger # before Eating	Time	Items/Amount	Hunger # after Eating

Thin Within Observations and Corrections Chart—Day 20

Observations	Day 20
1. I ate when my body was hungry.	
2. I ate in a calm environment by reducing distractions.	
3. I ate when I was sitting.	
4. I ate when my body and mind were relaxed.	
5. I ate and drank the things my body enjoyed.	
6. I paid attention to my food while eating.	
7. I ate slowly, savoring each bite.	
8. I stopped before my body was full.	

Part III
Enabled to Live Authentically and Abundantly

◌◌◌

Resisting No More

But for you who revere my name,
the sun of righteousness will rise with healing in its wings.
And you will go out and leap like calves released from the stall.
—Malachi 4:2

God releases captives, sets the prisoners free, gives sight to the blind, and binds up the broken-hearted. As we revere His name, we have the promise that we will go out and leap for joy in our newfound freedom!

Yesterday we purposed to fix our eyes on Jesus and to cast off the sin that so easily entangles us (Hebrews 12:2). We shook off the fetters of unforgiveness that had lain deep within the confines of our hearts. Now we emerge victorious from the clouds of desert dust. He leads us further still in a *triumphal procession in Christ and . . . spreads everywhere the fragrance of the knowledge of Him* (2 Corinthians 2:14). The *river whose streams make glad the city of our God* (Psalm 46:4) has washed over our parched hearts.

Our flesh machinery, our unworkable beliefs, and any thoughts raised up against the knowledge of God have been torn down. God has crushed strongholds that once stood like proud sentries over a heart, yet to be relinquished fully. We pray that you have surrendered to the Lord your heartache and pain, trusting that in His sovereignty He will redeem it. Truly it is only in knowing with confidence that He is sovereign and good that we can release our minds, our emotions, our wills, and our unmet needs to Him.

Over the past twenty days you have been involved in a restoration process. As you can see, it has been about much more than your physical "tent" or body. Truly, if you were to find yourself at the end of these thirty days smaller in size, yet without the peace, joy, and freedom we have been pursuing, it would all be in vain. *It is for freedom that Christ has set us free* (Galatians 5:1). He came that we might *have life, and have it abundantly* (John 10:10).

Most recently you were called upon to release anyone you had not forgiven.

It is our prayer that you persevered through that exercise and emerged truly blessed for having done so. As we humbly come to God, seeking His purposes and His plan, willing to be conformed to His character, we are perhaps more "real" than ever before. We are putting to death daily the deeds of the flesh, including the retaining of the false self or what Brennan Manning calls "the impostor." This is the person that we have presented to the public to gain approval, because we felt the need to look as if we had it all together.

According to Brennan Manning, "The impostor is attentive to the size, shape, and color of the bandages that veil my nothingness. The false self persuades me to be preoccupied with my weight. If I binge on a pint of Häagen-Dazs peanut butter vanilla and the scale signals distress the following morning, I am crestfallen. A beautiful day of sunshine beckons, but for the self-absorbed impostor, the bloom is off the rose. The minor vanities kidnap my attention away from the indwelling God and temporarily rob me of the joy of God's Holy Spirit. Yet the false self rationalizes my preoccupation with my waistline and overall appearance and whispers, 'A fat, sloppy image will diminish your credibility in ministry.' Cunning."[1]

As Manning points out, our flesh can easily dupe us. Dressed in the trappings of religious jargon, we try to justify our obsession with the outer man. It is only in surrendering our inner will fully to the Lord that we can begin to experience what it means to be *authentic* and live the holy life. Then we will no longer feel the need to pretend to be someone other than who God has made us to be. This is illustrated in figure 21-1.

This is what we mean by being thin *within*. It is authentically living on the outside what is genuinely present on the inside. Our desire is to have a heart in which Christ will dwell and be at home. As we allow Him to abide there and resolve to keep nothing from Him, He makes us more like Himself inside and out. The false or flesh life is crucified daily so that the Christlike life may shine through.

Jonathan Edwards, a great man of God who radically influenced the spiritual condition of the people early in our country's history, counted the cost of following our great God and King. Expressing his resolve to live set apart for the Lord, he wrote:

> I claim no right to myself—no right to this understanding, this will, these affections that are in me; neither do I have any right to this

body or its members—no right to this tongue, to these hands, feet, ears or eyes.

I have given myself clear away and not retained anything of my own. I have been to God this morning and told Him I have given myself wholly to Him. I have given every power, so that for the future I claim no right to myself in any respect. I have expressly promised Him, for by His grace I will not fail. I take Him as my whole portion and felicity; looking upon nothing else as any part of my happiness.[2]

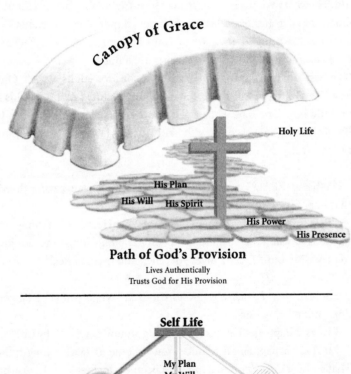

Path of God's Provision

Lives Authentically
Trusts God for His Provision

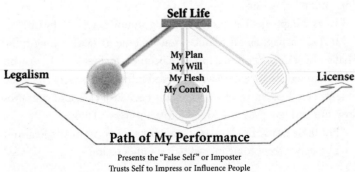

Path of My Performance

Presents the "False Self" or Imposter
Trusts Self to Impress or Influence People

figure 21–1

The release of "self" requires us to be responsible for our choices and actions. As Richard, a Thin Within participant, points out, "With freedom comes a responsibility to be honest with God and die to my demands. When I am honest, He meets me and true spiritual growth happens."

As we mature, we cease to blame others for our current behaviors or conditions. It means we choose how we will respond to what life brings—to what the Lord allows. We respond thoughtfully and prayerfully instead of reacting in our flesh.

The Lord created you, and He wants to shine forth through you to the world. He wants you to be real. It may be a frightening prospect, but it is wonderful to live authentically, to surrender all unto Him. He wants you to choose not to withhold any part of yourself from Him. He has plans for you—plans for good, not harm, a future and a hope.

The best children's stories offer many lessons for adults as well. One of these is *The Velveteen Rabbit*. It is a tale about a stuffed rabbit and his love for a little boy. One day, while on the nursery shelf with the other toys, Rabbit initiates a conversation with Skin Horse, who was "old and wise and experienced."

"What is REAL?" asked the Rabbit. "Does it mean having things that buzz inside you and a stick-out handle?"

"Real isn't how you are made," said the Skin Horse. "It's a thing that happens to you. When a child loves you for a long, long time, not just to play with, but REALLY loves you, then you become Real."

"Does it hurt?"

"Sometimes." For he was always truthful. "When you are Real you don't mind being hurt."

"Does it happen all at once, like being wound up, or bit by bit?"

"It doesn't happen all at once. You become. It takes a long time. That's why it doesn't often happen to people who break easily, or who have sharp edges, or who have to be carefully kept. Generally, by the time you are Real, most of your hair has been loved off, and your eyes drop out and you get loose in the joints and very shabby.

"But these things don't matter at all, because once you are Real you can't be ugly, except to people who don't understand."[3]

You are a precious child of God and you are on the path of becoming "real." It may be painful, but it is well worth the effort. You can never be ugly when you are real, "except to people who don't understand."

Take Action

Becoming "real" can be painful as we have learned throughout this building project. Yet by the grace of God it is in becoming real we discover that we have wings with which to fly. As you persevere in your efforts to be real, and to be a man or woman of God, consider for a moment the following questions:

+ What are ways that you have presented a "false self" or impostor to the world?

_____

_____

_____

+ Narrow the scope down a bit now. What are ways you have presented a "false self" or impostor to the world relative to your view of your body and your eating?

_____

_____

_____

When we surrender ourselves to the Lord, releasing our mind, will, emotions, and unmet needs, we begin truly to experience the abundant holy life. LaDonna, who struggled with various issues stemming from excessive abuse as a child explains, "I know all things are possible with God, and I have clung to Him and to His promises. He even helped me to overcome panic attacks that I experienced for so many years. I was then able to speak to a group of high school girls about overcoming anorexia and a negative self-image."

As LaDonna surrendered her unmet needs to the Lover of her soul, she became free to experience the joy of walking in the abundant life that Christ came to give her. Our gracious God redeemed her traumatic experiences, and used her to impact the lives of other women. Hopefully you have learned

a great deal in recent days about God's character and His plans for you as
you cooperate more fully with Him.

When the Israelites crossed the Jordan River, Joshua commanded twelve
men to gather stones from the middle of the riverbed and to place them on
dry ground as a reminder to future generations of how the Lord had delivered them and given them the land. We can follow this practice, honoring
the Lord for what we have seen Him do so far in our lives.

I have a friend who takes a large river rock and writes with a permanent
ink marker the date and way in which she has seen God's presence manifest
in her family's lives. One at a time, more rocks have been added to the col-
lection. The river rocks now adorn her garden, visible reminders of the ways
in which God has answered prayer, provided insight, delivered her from
sin—the list goes on and on. They are literal "memorial stones" of God's
incredible goodness and faithfulness.

Let's take stock of the miles you have traveled. In the chart below, record
what you have released to the care of God. Include a remembrance of how
you felt as you released it, and how you are feeling about it now.

What I Have Released	How I Felt about It at the Time	How I Feel about It Now

What are some ways that you can think of to remind yourself of God's goodness and faithfulness to you?

_____

_____

_____

From the opening verses in Genesis to the closing page of Revelation, there is no question that our God takes the initiative to dwell among us, extending Himself in a love relationship. From cover to cover, His Word breathes an invitation to our souls to draw near and to go deeper with Him. First John 4:19 says that we love God because He first loved us. In His love and grace He has taken the initiative to dwell within us. Loving Him is our response to His awesome overture.

For the remainder of our journey we pray that you will take time to write gratitude statements to God each day. This is something you might continue to do even after our journey together ends.

As we practice gratitude, we find ourselves not so focused on ourselves. As we turn our eyes toward God we experience the lifting up of our own spirits. On the lines below write at least ten things for which you have gratitude in your heart to God.

Gratitude List

_____

_____

_____

(Also consider establishing a "thanksgiving journal" as a memorial to God, honoring the wonderful work He has done in your life.)

Perhaps as you've written, you have been reminded of additional ways in which you can offer yourself specifically to God. Are there still recesses of your heart that have not been relinquished? Won't you take time to climb up into Abba's lap right now and offer them to Him? In the space below, write a prayer, sharing with Him your desire to do this, or simply record what you have yet to surrender to the Lover of your soul. He will help make your heart more willing to release it unto Him.

_____

_____

_____

_____

_____

How can we resist abandoning ourselves to such a wonderful God? Let's continue to put to death anything that remains of the false self that we have accepted for so long. Let's press on to become authentic in Christ by releasing ourselves into His incredible hands. As Hannah Whittall Smith has written:

> We mean an entire surrender of the whole being to God; spirit, soul, and body placed under His absolute control, for Him to do with us just what He pleases. We mean that the language of our soul, under all circumstances, and in view of every act, is to be, "Thy will be done." We mean the giving up of all liberty of choice. We mean a life of inevitable obedience. To a soul ignorant of God, this may look hard. But to those who know Him, it is the happiest and most restful of lives. He is our Father, and He loves us, and He knows just what is best, and therefore, of course, His will is the very most blessed thing that can come to us under all circumstances.[4]

Your Success Story

Did you have any new insights while you were reading today? Please record them below.

_____

_____

_____

Verses to Ponder

Though you have not seen him, you love him; and even though you do not see him now, you believe in him and are filled with an inexpressible and glorious joy, for you are receiving the goal of your faith, the salvation of your souls (1 Peter 1:8–9).

Give thanks in all circumstances, for this is God's will for you in Christ Jesus (1 Thessalonians 5:18).

Let the word of Christ dwell in you richly as you teach and admonish one another with all wisdom, and as you sing psalms, hymns and spiritual songs with gratitude in your hearts to God. And whatever you do, whether in word or deed, do it all in the name of the Lord Jesus, giving thanks to God the Father through him (Colossians 3:16–17).

Prayer

Dear Lord, thank You for the healing work You've done in my heart over the past twenty days. I praise You because Your works are wonderful. I know that every change that has taken place has been because of Your grace poured out, pressed down, and overflowing. Thank You that through Your Spirit I can put to death my "false self" and trust You more and more with my mind, will, emotions, and unmet needs. Help me to surrender myself more fully unto You, Lord, to be authentic and as I continue on this journey. In Jesus' name, Amen.

Medical Moment

Interestingly in this era of unparalleled scientific advances, there is a renewed interest in the relationship between faith and healing. More and more medical schools are offering courses in spirituality, and the medical literature is increasingly acknowledging the role of faith and prayer in influencing conditions as diverse as cardiac surgery and childhood leukemia. Such studies are difficult to devise and control, but a careful reading of such studies has convinced me of the validity of the conclusion. In this day of polypharmacy (a pill for everything) and the alarming increase in the incidence of adverse drug reactions, it is wonderful to recognize the effectiveness (with no negative side effects) of prayer as a valuable adjunct in the healing arts.

—ARTHUR HALLIDAY, M.D.

Success Tools

+ Fill in the Hunger Graph.
+ Fill in the Thin Within Food Log.
+ Use the Thin Within Observations and Corrections Chart for today.
+ Use the Thin Within Keys to Conscious Eating.

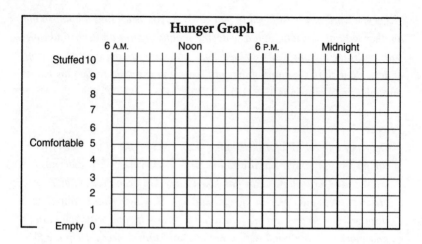

Thin Within Food Log

Hunger # before Eating	Time	Items/Amount	Hunger # after Eating

Thin Within Observations and Corrections Chart—Day 21

Observations	Day 21
1. I ate when my body was hungry.	
2. I ate in a calm environment by reducing distractions.	
3. I ate when I was sitting.	
4. I ate when my body and mind were relaxed.	
5. I ate and drank the things my body enjoyed.	
6. I paid attention to my food while eating.	
7. I ate slowly, savoring each bite.	
8. I stopped before my body was full.	

Thin Within Wisdom

God takes the initiative to dwell among us, extending Himself in a love relationship,

NOTES

1. Excerpted from *Abba's Child—The Cry of the Heart for Intimate Belonging* by Brennan Manning © 1994. Used by permission of NavPress Publishing Group. www.navpress.com. All rights reserved.
2. Jonathan Edwards.
3. Margery Williams, *The Velveteen Rabbit* (New York, New York: Random House, Inc., 1985), 8–10.
4. Hannah Whitall Smith.

❦

Confident of His Touch: Part 1

Be on your guard;
stand firm in the faith;
be men of courage;
be strong.
Do everything in love.
—1 Corinthians 16:13–14

The temple is nearing completion, though our finishing work will continue in the days remaining. We are building block upon block with the Master. We discussed in Day Fourteen the power of our beliefs. Today we will go a step further by seeking to conform our beliefs to the Word of God. Each block that we extract from the quarry of His Word will be placed carefully upon the foundation and nestled within the infrastructure to become part of a glorious temple, firm, steadfast, and immovable.

As we proceed along our walk of faith, hopefully your beliefs will have changed to reflect your greater confidence in God and your gratitude for all He is doing in your life. No longer does Romans 8:28 seem like a mere platitude: *And we know that in all things God works for the good of those who love him, who have been called according to his purpose.* Philip Yancey says that, "The Greek original text is more properly translated as follows, 'In everything that happens, God works for good with those who love him.'"[1]

We have seen that although not everything in life is good, God will walk with us through those trying times and He can turn it into good. Someone has said that when considering the ingredients of a delicious chocolate cake, it would be horrid trying to eat four cups of flour. Two cups of sugar would probably be quite sickening. Unsweetened chocolate is bitter to taste. Real butter would be tough to "stomach" by itself. To eat raw eggs would be disgusting and no longer even safe. And baking powder? Blah. However, when the Master Chef mixes these ingredients together, adding just the right amount of heat for the proper length of time, a wonderful delicacy emerges.

The trials and challenges of our lives work together in a similar way. Each one in isolation is unpleasant and undesirable. Some are downright disgusting. But in the Master Chef's hands all our trials can be turned into something sensational. Carmen, another Thin Within participant, shares her experience: "A lot of baggage came up and out as I realized how I had grieved the Lord by having food and weight take center stage. After the forgiveness exercises I felt renewed in my walk with the Lord. It brought healing in my relationship with Him."

During the past twenty-one days we have come face to face with our struggles, our failures, our sins, and our heartaches. But we have seen the hand of our great God in the midst of it all. He has shown us that He is forming all of our experiences into one great blessing. He is cooking up something fabulous.

God can use our struggle with compulsive overeating and our inappropriate view of our bodies to form and shape our character. To use another analogy, consider the underside of a tapestry where all sorts of loose threads are going every which way with no rhyme or reason. To us it looks like a big mess. However, on the topside, from God's perspective, we discover a perfect masterpiece from the hand of the Creator. Our lives are the same. The view from below appears chaotic at times but from above, He is weaving a wondrous design that will take our breath away.

On our journey so far we have come to see that our God is trustworthy. He wastes nothing. He weaves our trials, our sins, and our failures into the tapestry of our life to work for our ultimate good. It doesn't mean that He condones our sin or that He planned our failures or our wounding, but by His incredible grace He will use it all. The results will be amazing.

We can continue to trust in our God. As we believe in Him, He will be faithful. Our beliefs are very important, as we have already seen, because they lay the foundation for our behavior. In the next exercise, we will take some specific steps adapted from Dr. Charles Stanley to strengthen your belief system.

Steps to Strengthening Your Belief System

1. State with confidence and boldness: "God has equipped me with everything I need to be what He wants me to be and to accomplish what He wants me to accomplish."
2. Remind yourself often of the Lord's promise to make a way when there seems to be no way.

3. Highlight verses in your Bible that deal with courage, confidence, faith, and believing.
4. Pray the promises of God.
5. Visualize and affirm your assets.
6. Make and memorize a list of character qualities that you desire to develop.
7. Actively replace negative thoughts and statements with positive thoughts and statements.
8. When an obstacle arises, state boldly, "If God is for me, who can be against me?"
9. When you are feeling harassed by Satan, say aloud, "Father, God, I want to thank you that you are greater in me than anything Satan can do to me."
10. Remind yourself continually: "God is with me in this. He will never leave me or forsake me."[2]

Take Action

Today and tomorrow we will be focusing on Dr. Stanley's steps to strengthening our beliefs. On the last day of *Thin Within*, we will have the chance to stand back and appraise the work that has been done. It is our desire that you have a tool chest, ready to use as you continue to apply yourself to the maintenance of His temple—your soul, mind and body—in the days to follow.

1. **State with confidence and boldness: "God has equipped me with everything I need to be what He wants me to be and to accomplish what He wants me to accomplish."**

This step comes directly from scripture. Second Peter 1:3 says, *His divine power has given us everything we need for life and godliness through our knowledge of him who called us by his own glory and goodness.*

Take this scripture and personalize it. We have offered an example as follows.

God has given me, (your name), the power by His Holy Spirit so that I have all I need to make godly choices about food, eating, and my body. As I get to know more of His glory and goodness, I become more able to live my life through Him.

In the exercise below, you can personalize the scriptures as you apply them to your temple-refurbishing project.

Romans 8:1–2 (Look it up, then write your personalization here)

_____

_____

_____

Psalm 27:1

_____

_____

_____

Philippians 4:13

_____

_____

_____

You can personalize any verse in the Bible. This is a great way of experiencing God's Word coming alive in your life. Doing so will bolster your faith and strengthen your belief system.

2. **Remind yourself often of the Lord's promise to make a way when there seems to be no way.**

Whenever you find yourself feeling backed up against a wall, you can refer to your gratitude statements or your thanksgiving journal. There will be times when you are tempted to overeat. We hope those times will soon be fewer and farther between, but if and when they do come, we recommend reading Scripture as well as what you have written. What better way to be reminded that God always makes a way than by remembering and praising Him for what He has already done during your Thin Within journey. This will give you a fresh sense of God's plan and purpose for you.

Right now refer to any of the gratitude statements that you have written over the past few days. In the space below, bring each of the things before God, affirming that you know He is in control of even that which seems impossible. We have an example for you.

Dear Lord, I thank You that You have touched my heart so tenderly in the last few days. You have given me a willingness to forgive _____ and that is a miracle. If You can do that, You can do anything. Lord, You have also given me the strength to eat 0 to 5 and for that I am grateful. I know that You can

*help me with the temptation I have right now to order a take out pizza. Lord,
I am not hungry and I have dinner planned. I know that my desire for that
pizza is only due to my level of frustration right now. To eat the pizza would
be giving into the lust of my flesh. So I place my trust in You and pray for godly
patience. In Jesus' name, Amen.*

Now it is your turn.

_____

_____

_____

_____

3. Highlight verses in your Bible that deal with courage, confidence, faith, and believing.

In the back of your Bible you will most likely find a concordance that
lists many of the words found in your Bible. You can begin by finding a
verse for "courage." We suggest that you read at least a few verses before and
after each of the references, so you can understand the proper context for
that verse. After reading, we hope you will journal about the insights God
gave you.

In our Bible concordance, the first verse that refers to courage actually
uses the word "courageous," and it is found in Deuteronomy 31:6: *Be strong
and courageous. Do not be afraid or terrified because of them, for the* LORD
your God goes with you; he will never leave you nor forsake you.

If I were to journal this verse I might say something like this, "Lord, thank
You that You give me strength and courage to face my daily challenges. I
don't need to find comfort in the empty arms of food any longer. You are
with me and will never forsake me. What a great, glorious God You are."

You can highlight all of the verses you find and/or record them in your
journal. This is a wonderful learning experience and can be an insightful
chronicling of your journey of faith. On the lines below, write two of the
verses and what they mean to you.

_____

_____

_____

_____

4. Pray the promises of God.

This is a powerful tool, packed with the strength and might of the Lord Almighty. Amazing things happen when we pray God's word. When you are doing this for the first time, you may find it especially helpful to use scripture that was written as a prayer. (For instance, Ephesians 1:16–23; 3:14–21, or many of the Psalms.)

Therefore, I urge you, brothers, in view of God's mercy, to offer your bodies as living sacrifices, holy and pleasing to God—this is your spiritual act of worship. Do not conform any longer to the pattern of this world, but be transformed by the renewing of your mind. Then you will be able to test and approve what God's will is—his good, pleasing and perfect will (Romans 12:1–2).

You might pray by saying something like this: *Lord, You have been so merciful to me. Therefore, I want to give myself totally to You as an offering. I pray that You will find my offering pleasing and holy, Lord. I worship You today with my choices. This will include when I start and when I stop eating. Please renew my mind so that I, (your name), can know Your good, pleasing, and perfect will.*

Look up each of the following verses and then write out a prayer using the ideas that you glean from each scripture.

1 John 4:4

_____

_____

_____

_____

Psalm 20:4–5

_____

_____

_____

_____

As we discussed on Day Fifteen, God wants to be a part of the minute details of our lives. Praying scripture brings honor to Him and releases His power in your life.

For more ideas on scriptures to pray, turn to the Psalms.

5. Visualize and affirm your assets.

Many Christians are apprehensive about using the tool of visualization. This is understandable because it is often used inappropriately. However, if you remember that Christ made use of parables, and if you consider that a parable is a word picture, we can see that godly visualizations are to be found throughout the pages of the New Testament.

This is also seen in the Old Testament where the prophet Nathan used imagery to confront David about his adultery with Bathsheba and the murder of Uriah. He did so by painting a mental image in David's mind first (2 Samuel 12). Nathan knew that God would work through David's mind to affect his beliefs about his sin and the forthcoming confession. This is how Nathan was able to prompt David's repentant actions and their subsequent results. (Remember Day Fourteen?)

In order to make godly use of the visualization tool, which has been used by the devil and the world for ungodly purposes, it must first be rooted in God's purposes for us. As we indicated in Days Three and Sixteen, God's purposes for us are to glorify Him and to be conformed to the image of His Son. So visualizations are appropriate, but only when they are aligned with God's will and His Word.

Turn now to your goals in Day Sixteen. As you recall, we encouraged you to seek the wisdom of God for your goals so they would be in accordance with His will. You restated your goals and then broke each goal into workable pieces. Having goals is an asset. In fact, you may have heard it said, the person who aims at nothing is sure to hit it every time. Having no goals is a liability.

Read goal #1 from Day Sixteen. Close your eyes for a minute and picture yourself cooperating with God in the goal you have listed. Picture, too, the peace and joy that fills your life as you realize this goal in your mind. Record your impressions here:

_____

_____

Read goal #2 from Day Sixteen. Visualize yourself actually accomplishing the goal. Afterward, record your impressions here.

_____

_____

Do the same with goal #3.

_____

_____

To further affirm any additional assets He has given you, thank God for a heart that is willing to participate with Him. Praise Him for the support of any godly person that has come alongside of you. The body of Christ is one of our richest assets. For what other assets can you visualize, affirm, and praise God?

_____

_____

_____

Today we are reinforcing the work done during the first twenty-one days of our building project as well as catching a glimpse for the future. Our minds are transformed when we allow them to be renewed by God's Word of truth. Please do not view these suggestions as a legalistic list of dos and don'ts that you must follow to be successful. This is offered to you as a resource for a constant supply of the living water that can slake any thirst and of the bread of life that causes us never to hunger.

Today we have focused on five of ten ways of strengthening our faith or belief systems. Tomorrow we will focus on the other five. It is our prayer that you are experiencing joy and satisfaction as you continue with this process. Your labor has not been in vain. Keep up the good work!

Your Success Story

Record any new insights you had while reading today.

_____

_____

_____

Verses to Ponder

I have been crucified with Christ and I no longer live, but Christ lives in me. The life I live in the body, I live by faith in the Son of God, who loved me and gave himself for me (Galatians 2:20).

We live by faith, not by sight (2 Corinthians 5:7).

In him and through faith in him we may approach God with freedom and confidence (Ephesians 3:12).

Prayer

Dear Lord, thank You that You are always with me, sustaining my faith by Your grace and by Your Holy Spirit. Lord, I pray that I will have a greater desire not only to read Your Word but to allow it to be written on the tablet of my heart. As I meditate on Scripture, cause it to satisfy my soul, I pray that Your Holy Spirit will encourage me to walk in the confidence of who I am in Christ and that I may continue making progress as You restore my body, the temple in which You dwell. In Jesus' precious name, Amen.

Medical Moment

Sadly Americans get far too little exercise. Our sedentary jobs, push-button lives, and spectator recreational activities are major contributors to the burgeoning of our weight. It is estimated that insufficient exercise is linked to at least seventeen chronic diseases that cause 250,000 deaths annually and cost $2 trillion to treat. It is extremely difficult to release weight solely by exercising. The reason for this is the incredible efficiency of the body. For a 125-pound person to lose one pound, he or she would have to run for five hours, or bicycle for seven hours, or swim for seven and a half hours, or jog for eight hours, or walk for fourteen hours. This is unrealistic for most of us and something we don't recommend.

The good news is that exercise is very good for us in a variety of ways. It relieves stress, improves skin, increases bone density, and muscle mass. Exercise gives us more energy and an increased sense of emotional and psychological well-being. Exercise helps us determine our true hunger signals and it is a marvelous adjunct for weight reduction when you eat according to your God-given hunger-fullness sensations. We recommend the keys to conscious eating plus regular daily exercise (approximately thirty minutes). Choose something that you enjoy doing so that you will continue doing it. You will be thrilled with the ongoing results.

—Arthur Halliday, M.D.

Success Tools

- ✦ Fill in the Hunger Graph.
- ✦ Fill in the Thin Within Food Log.
- ✦ Use the Thin Within Observations and Corrections Chart for today.
- ✦ Use the Thin Within Keys to Conscious Eating.
- ✦ Use the Gratitude List or your Thanksgiving Journal to record what you are thankful for today.

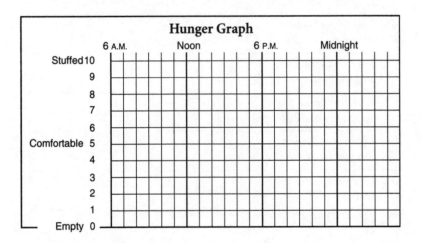

Thin Within Food Log

Hunger # before Eating	Time	Items/Amount	Hunger # after Eating

Thin Within Observations and Corrections Chart—Day 22

Observations	Day 22
1. I ate when my body was hungry.	
2. I ate in a calm environment by reducing distractions.	
3. I ate when I was sitting.	
4. I ate when my body and mind were relaxed.	
5. I ate and drank the things my body enjoyed.	
6. I paid attention to my food while eating.	
7. I ate slowly, savoring each bite.	
8. I stopped before my body was full.	

Gratitude List

_____

_____

_____

Thin Within Wisdom

Use some of the tools we covered today to begin to build your life in a fresh way.

NOTES

1. Philip Yancey, *Reaching for the Invisible God* (Grand Rapids, Michigan: Zondervan, 2000), 59.
2. Charles Stanley, *Success God's Way* (Nashville, Tennessee: Thomas Nelson Publishers, 2000), 211–213.

Confident of His Touch: Part 2

Abram believed the LORD, and he credited it to him as righteousness.
—Genesis 15:6

Your life is beginning to stand as a tribute to what God can do when one is given over to the Lord. We pray that the glory of God is beginning to be more evident in you. Do you see it? Praise Him, for He has begun a good work within you!

With only a week left in our project, let us be doubly diligent about applying ourselves to the work of God in building His temple. We have come far and have accomplished much in the strength that only His grace can give. As Acts 20:24 reminds us, *I consider my life worth nothing to me, if only I may finish the race and complete the task the Lord Jesus has given me —the task of testifying to the gospel of God's grace.*

Yesterday we elaborated on the first five of Charles Stanley's "Steps to Strengthening Your Belief System." Take a minute to record any additional thoughts you may have before we move on.

_____

_____

_____

It may take some practice to feel comfortable utilizing a new tool, as some tools are more effective than others. Debbie, a graduate of Thin Within, was considering what enabled her to maintain her natural God-given size. She states, "The Hunger Graphs and eating from 0 to 5 are important, as well as prayer and Bible study." However, you will discover that, when it comes to building and maintaining God's beautiful temple, nothing is quite so effective as the tool of faith, supported by a good strong dose of His Word.

Do your best to present yourself to God as one approved, a workman who does not need to be ashamed and who correctly handles the word of truth (2 Timothy 2:15).

Now let's review Charles Stanley's suggested steps to a stronger faith.

Steps to Strengthening Your Belief System

1. State with confidence and boldness: "God has endowed me with everything I need to be what He wants me to be and to accomplish what He wants me to accomplish."
2. Remind yourself often of the Lord's promise to make a way when there seems to be no way.
3. Highlight verses in your Bible that deal with courage, confidence, faith, and believing.
4. Pray the promises of God.
5. Visualize and affirm your assets.
6. Make and memorize a list of character qualities that you desire to develop.
7. Actively replace negative thoughts and statements with positive thoughts and statements.
8. When an obstacle arises, state boldly, "If God is for me, who can be against me?"
9. When you are feeling harassed by Satan, say aloud, "Father, God, I want to thank you that you are greater in me than anything Satan can do to me."
10. Remind yourself continually: "God is with me in this. He will never leave me or forsake me."[1]

A rebuilding task of this magnitude requires more than a mallet and chisel. The following tools will enable you to build even more efficiently and reliably. Let's familiarize ourselves with the last five steps to strengthening your beliefs.

Take Action

6. Make and memorize a list of character qualities that you desire to develop.

The following is a list of some of the character qualities described in Scripture:

Believing	Blameless	Bold	Cheerful
Compassionate	Comforting	Courageous	Content
Diligent	Discerning	Disciplined	Encouraging
Enduring	Exemplary	Faithful	Fervent

Forbearing	Forgiving	Friendly	Fruitful
Gentle	Giving	Godly	Gracious
Grounded	Happy	Holy	Honest

As you can see, this only covers the first part of the alphabet. The list goes on and on. Take a moment in prayer right now to ask the Lord what character qualities He wants to develop in you. You can use anything in this list or ask Him to supply others that might be more relevant. List three character traits that you feel are in line with His purposes for you.

1. _____
2. _____
3. _____

Now visualize what each of these might look like in your life. Include any ways in which that character trait would impact your relationship with food, your body, and the Lord. Record your answers on the lines below.

Character trait #1 is to be

_____

I would like to incorporate this in my life in the following ways:

_____

_____

Character trait #2 is to be

_____

I would like to incorporate this in my life in the following ways:

_____

_____

Character trait #3 is to be

_____

I would like to incorporate this in my life in the following ways:

_____

_____

Can you see how incorporating these character traits will add strength and power to your godly temple? Be assured that they will.

7. **Actively replace negative thoughts and statements with positive thoughts and statements.**

On Day Eleven you identified some of the false beliefs or lies that may have contributed to problems with food and eating. Step #7 offers a way of taking captive, in the present moment, any inappropriate thoughts *before* they take you captive.

Cheryl writes, "The Thin Within principles apply to every area of my life. I learned to renew my mind with biblically positive messages and to replace the negative ones. At first I struggled with saying positive things about my body. Even though my legs were fat, I said, 'Thank you, God, for my legs, which have taken me so many places over all these years.'" Cheryl learned the value of replacing her negative false thoughts with positive true thoughts.

Negative Thoughts to Replace	Positive Thought to Replace It
I can't seem to stop at a 5 on the hunger scale. I am just a hopeless failure.	The hunger graph is a tool to help me to observe and correct. I will press on and pray for God's power to equip me to observe and correct, to repent at those times when I am willful. I know I am *not* a hopeless failure. Today with Christ I will do it. Philippians 4:13
Your turn:	

✦ In the left-hand column in the graph on page 246, identify any negative thoughts that you have about yourself, your body, food, or even other people—anything at all. Ask God to reveal other negative thoughts of which you may not be aware. In the column on the right, replace the negative thought with a positive one. To apply this activity personally and make it a part of your thinking, it would be helpful to pray as you work. Specifically confess to God the negative thought in the left column and tell Him that you now choose to replace that negative thought with the positive one based on the truth of His Word in the right column. Become aware of any runaway thoughts and take them captive to the obedience of Christ by using this technique. An example is done for you.

8. **When an obstacle arises, state boldly, "If God is for me, who can be against me?"**

To help you utilize this step we suggest memorizing the following scripture:

What, then, shall we say in response to this? If God is for us, who can be against us? He who did not spare his own Son, but gave him up for us all—how will he not also, along with him, graciously give us all things? (Romans 8:31–32)

This is just one powerful tool that you can use in the restoring of your body, soul, mind, and heart—God's temple. The Bible encourages us to tuck the Word of truth away in our hearts so that we receive its blessings and benefits moment by moment.

How can a young man keep his way pure? By living according to your word. I seek you with all my heart; do not let me stray from your commands. I have hidden your word in my heart that I might not sin against you (Psalm 119:9–11).

There are many different ways of incorporating scriptural truths into our daily lives. Whatever your approach, if you face an obstacle that seems insurmountable, you can remind yourself, "If God is for me, who can be against me?"

9. **When you are feeling harassed by Satan, say aloud, "Father, God, I want to thank you that you are greater in me than anything Satan can do to me."**

Thanking God for the truths offered in Scripture is a valuable exercise in bolstering your faith, especially when the enemy of your soul confronts you.

It is important to maintain godly boundaries for the temple of God and the indwelling Holy Spirit. All of His power and presence are available within you *to will and to act according to His good purpose* (Philippians 2:13).

List some situations or circumstances in which you find yourself feeling most harassed by the Enemy:

_____

_____

_____

When these situations arise, refute the harassment of the Enemy with this simple truth from 1 John 4:4:

You, dear children, are from God and have overcome them, because the one who is in you is greater than the one who is in the world.

10. **Remind yourself continually: "God is with me in this. He will never leave me or forsake me."**[1]

In the garden of Eden the serpent's primary weapon was the seed of doubt that he carefully planted in Adam and Eve's minds about the character of God. But the truth is that God is faithful. He is "omnipresent," meaning that He is everywhere present and always with you. You can't run away from Him—even if you try.

Where can I go from your Spirit? Where can I flee from your presence? If I go up to the heavens, you are there; if I make my bed in the depths, you are there. If I rise on the wings of the dawn, if I settle on the far side of the sea, even there your hand will guide me, your right hand will hold me fast (Psalm 139:7–10).

Isn't that reassuring? God will not abandon you as you wrestle with issues of food and weight, even if you "fail" with 0 to 5 eating. He is still with you, loving you, calling you to return to Him so He can wipe the tears from your eyes and lead you down the path of His provision as you live the holy life. When the enemy asks, "Where is your God?" resolutely declare, "He is in the same place He has always been. He is right here with me."

God has said, "Never will I leave you; never will I forsake you" (Hebrews 13:5b).

In figure 23-1, we have illustrated the characteristics of both paths. The surest way to return to the path of God's provision is by repentance. As we observe, we identify the truth about our behavior and agree with God that a correction is in order. We then confess the truth we observe, and identify the faulty thinking and fleshly behaviors. He further places within us a desire to make the godly correction. This is repentance, and it results in returning to the path of God's provision where we are filled with peace, joy, and rest.

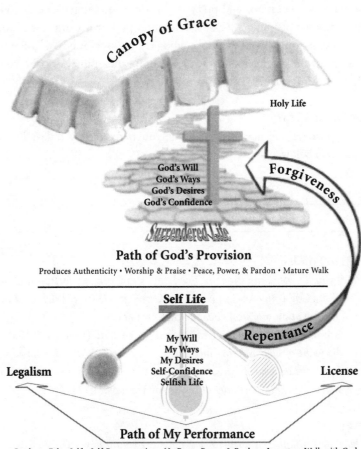

figure 23–1

If you discover you have an unforgiving heart as we discussed on Day Twenty, you can do the same thing: repent first, allowing the Lord to establish a forgiving heart. In the power of a prayer, in the stillness of a moment, you will find that God waits to extend His grace. His compassions are never ending. Return to Him, admitting your need for Him as He enfolds you in His arms and cleanses your heart. In His mercy and grace, He restores a right spirit within you (1 Peter 5:10).

In His Word the Lord has promised to remain with you and in you forever.

You are now equipped and prepared to continue maintenance of your body, God's temple, long after our restoration project is complete. If you apply these steps now, while the rebuilding is still under way, you will ultimately realize a greatly reinforced foundation and framework for your body, mind, and spirit.

Your Success Story

Did you have any new insights while you were reading today? Please record them below.

_____

_____

_____

Verses to Ponder

I love you, O Lord, my strength. The Lord is my rock, my fortress and my deliverer; my God is my rock, in whom I take refuge. He is my shield and the horn of my salvation, my stronghold (Psalm 18:1–2).

Your word is a lamp to my feet and a light for my path (Psalm 119:105).

For the word of God is living and active. Sharper than any double-edged sword, it penetrates even to dividing soul and spirit, joints and marrow; it judges the thoughts and attitudes of the heart (Hebrews 4:12).

Prayer

Dear Lord, thank You for all You supply as I continue with You on the path of Your provision and restoration. I am so thankful that Your strength equips me to persevere in the face of my own willful rebellion, the lies from the Enemy, and the weakness of my own flesh. Thank You, Lord, that I can confess my wrongdoing when I go my own way, repent, and turn back to You. I praise You, Lord, that You are the restorer of my soul and that You will help me surrender all to You so that I can experience the holy abundant life. In Jesus' name, Amen.

Medical Moment

For some time Christians have known that prayer and faith "work." However, there is a new "renaissance" in the medical community where science is beginning to take note of the fact that faith and prayer seem to have an impact on the health and healing of patients. Some remain skeptical, of course. But there can be little doubt that those with a practicing faith experience fewer troubles with high blood pressure, stress-related maladies, drug abuse, and alcoholism. People who have faith tend to recover more readily when they are taken ill, and heart disease, cancer, and depression don't seem to have quite the death grip on people who pray diligently. Whether science will ever "prove" it or not, we know that our God is great and that our belief in Him and His transforming power in our life makes a huge difference. As we trust in Him, we experience joy, peace, and contentment. These cannot be measured, but they cannot help but have a positive effect on all aspects of our life.

—ARTHUR HALLIDAY, M.D.

Success Tools

+ Fill in the Hunger Graph.
+ Fill in the Thin Within Food Log.
+ Use the Thin Within Observations and Corrections Chart for today.
+ Use the Thin Within Keys to Conscious Eating.
+ Use the Gratitude List or your Thanksgiving Journal to record what you are thankful for today.

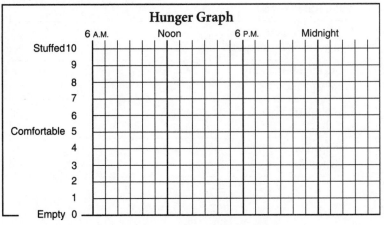

Thin Within Food Log

Hunger # before Eating	Time	Items/Amount	Hunger # after Eating

Thin Within Observations and Corrections Chart—Day 23

Observations	Day 23
1. I ate when my body was hungry.	
2. I ate in a calm environment by reducing distractions.	
3. I ate when I was sitting.	
4. I ate when my body and mind were relaxed.	
5. I ate and drank the things my body enjoyed.	
6. I paid attention to my food while eating.	
7. I ate slowly, savoring each bite.	
8. I stopped before my body was full.	

Gratitude List

_____

_____

_____

Thin Within Wisdom

A little at a time—that is how incredible monuments are built! So, too your life.

NOTE

1. Charles Stanley, *Success God's Way* (Nashville, Tennessee: Thomas Nelson Publishers, 2000), 211–213.

To Run and Not Grow Weary

But those who hope in the LORD will renew their strength.
They will soar on wings like eagles;
they will run and not grow weary,
they will walk and not be faint.
—Isaiah 40:31

Walking the path of God's provision, we discover that life in the Lord is an adventure. We continue to see the handiwork of God displayed at each turn. The challenges we confront are opportunities for us to see the hand of God clearly revealed.

His grace imparts hope into every moment. As we hope in Him and in His strength, we experience the renewal that we so vitally need. Once again we stretch out our wings and experience the lift beneath them provided by the winds of His grace. As Isaiah 40 says, our strength is renewed as we wait on Him. And as we walk the walk of faith, we have no cause to faint—because His grace continues to nourish our spirits! Our God is most assuredly in control, which is affirmed throughout the pages of the Bible.

Two related truths appear repeatedly in God's Word. First, as His children we will be tested. Job is an example of this biblical truth. However, even in the testing of Job, Satan displayed no power that was not first permitted by God and used for God's express purposes (Job 42:1).

Second, as difficult as it may be for us to swallow, the truth is that the most effective forming and shaping of our character takes place during times of suffering.

We also rejoice in our sufferings, because we know that suffering produces perseverance; perseverance, character; and character, hope. And hope does not disappoint us, because God has poured out his love into our hearts by the Holy Spirit, whom he has given us (Romans 5:3–5).

There is a distinct link between perseverance and the development of character. A similar link exists between character and a sense of hope. Few have known this as well as Simon Peter, who was transformed by God's hand through suffering. Some of his sufferings came about, of course, because of his own sin (most notably his denial of Christ). Just before predicting Peter's denial, Jesus revealed something else very intriguing:

Simon, Simon, Satan has asked to sift you as wheat (Luke 22:31).

Some of Peter's sufferings came about because the Lord granted Satan the right to test or "sift" him. It happened then as it does now. Candace, who continues to release weight on the way to her natural God-given size, describes her experience: "As the Lord has healed me of the wounds of my past, I am amazed to see how much of the suffering and sin He has taken from my life and formed character qualities that are more like Christ.

"I never would have clung to Christ so much, never would have hungered for His Word," Candace continues, "if I hadn't been 'afflicted' as David describes in the Psalms. He truly has taken everything I considered ugly and used it for good. I know I am stronger in Him and more tenderhearted and compassionate as a result of the trials I have gone through over the past thirty years. It hasn't been easy, but I see that God had something far greater in mind for me as His purpose and His plan was being perfected."

Nothing can come to us unless He allows it. Jesus told Peter about the request of the Enemy and provided him with confident assurance and a commission:

But I have prayed for you, Simon, that your faith may not fail. And when you have turned back, strengthen your brothers (Luke 22:32).

Somehow, through this experience of testing and "turning back," Peter's faith was increased so that he could be used by God to strengthen others. An amazing thing happened on the day of Pentecost (Acts 2:14–40). Peter was the first to stand up and give one of the most compelling sermons ever delivered! The results speak for themselves.

Those who accepted his message were baptized, and about three thousand were added to their number that day (Acts 2:41).

Satan asked Jesus if he could sift Peter. Jesus countered by praying for Peter, who repented of his denial of Christ and reaffirmed his commitment to Christ. Peter was then told to feed His sheep (John 21:15–18).

After his trials and suffering and the subsequent outpouring of the Holy Spirit at Pentecost, Peter's character was changed forever. He was no longer ashamed of Christ. Instead, risking life and limb, he boldly stepped forward and proclaimed that salvation could be found only in Jesus. Later, to benefit and strengthen other weary sheep, he wrote:

Now for a little while you may have had to suffer grief in all kinds of trials. These have come so that your faith—of greater worth than gold, which perishes even though refined by fire—may be proved genuine and may result in praise, glory and honor when Jesus Christ is revealed (1 Peter 1:6–7).

Peter knew what it was like to be tested in the crucible of life, having experienced the Refiner's fire. He became convinced that God was in control, even in the volatile political climate of his day. In fact, Peter wrote these very words to those who, because of the persecution of believers, had been scattered throughout the Mediterranean world.

Paul also encouraged people not to remain focused on the troubles of this world. He wrote, *For what is seen is temporary, but what is unseen is eternal.* He assured his readers, *Our light and momentary troubles are achieving for us an eternal glory that far outweighs them all* (2 Corinthians 4:17–18). In fact, the theme of rejoicing in trials and testing reoccurs throughout the entire living Word of God. James also taught accordingly:

Consider it pure joy, my brothers, whenever you face trials of many kinds, because you know that the testing of your faith develops perseverance. Perseverance must finish its work so that you may be mature and complete, not lacking anything (James 1:2–4).

In order to be made mature and complete in our faith, we will undergo trials. But we can know without a doubt that the Lord is in control. He intends that anything we experience be used for our growth and our good, achieving for us an "eternal glory."

Can this apply to your body's restoration as the temple of the Holy Spirit? Yes, it can. Throughout Scripture we read about incidents when food was used by the Enemy to distract God's people from His purposes and plans. In Genesis, the fall of man is linked to a lust for a forbidden fruit, which fell outside of God's boundaries for His children. Later Esau sold his birthright to Jacob for the sake of food he wanted immediately. The Israelites saw the glory of the Lord during the plagues of Egypt, the parting of the Red Sea, and as He personally led them day and night through the desert. Still, partly due to discontentment with being fed the same food from heaven each day, they forgot what slavery was really like, griping instead about God's desert "menu":

If only we had died by the LORD's hand in Egypt. There we sat round pots of meat and ate all the food we wanted, but you have brought us out into this desert to starve this entire assembly to death (Exodus 16:3).

An unholy lust for food is central to these incidents, found in the first two books of the Bible. Others are apparent throughout God's Word. Thankfully, whatever temptations the world, the flesh, and the devil can use, God supersedes to build character and strength in His people.

It is very possible that you may find yourself undergoing trials, sufferings, and temptations with regard to food and eating. As Mary Kate, another workshop participant said, "I know God makes a way of escape when I turn to him. And loving Him means obeying Him. My favorite verse to apply to my struggle with eating is 1 Corinthians 10:13, *No temptation has overtaken you but such as is common to man; and God is faithful, who will not allow you to be tempted beyond what you are able, but with the temptation will provide the way of escape also, that you may be able to endure it"* (NASB).

Your resolve to finish the restoration and subsequent maintenance of your body, God's temple, will undoubtedly be challenged; so be prepared and well armed. Look on your trials as an opportunity for the Lord to form and shape your character. He will provide a way of escape if you are open to it. You can be confident that He will not allow anything to prevent the accomplishment of His plan and purpose for His beloved, *you.* He will provide the grace and the strength you need to emerge victorious.

Dear reader, we know this with confidence only because of our own experiences with trials and testing. It has only been after many years of hardships that we have learned that God always has greater purposes in store than those we can see at the time. We can turn to and rest in His tender mercies, and His amazing grace.

Take a moment and ask God for wisdom. Then answer these questions: "What must I do to complete the restoration project God has begun in me? How have I been tested and challenged?"

_____

_____

_____

_____

There are many ways in which Thin Within participants have experienced testing. We encourage you to persevere when faced with the following:

1. **A Test of Obedience:** Press on and be willing to experience hunger. Don't lose sight of the goal.

2. **A Test of Freedom:** Stay in present time. Don't allow your past to dictate how you will respond in the present moment.

3. **A Test of Belief:** Continue to take captive unworkable beliefs.

4. **A Test of Faith:** Observe and correct, allowing the grace of God to guide you into the obedient life of holiness.

5. **A Test of Perseverance:** Persevere. Don't give up. Continue to press on.

6. **A Test of Tenderness:** Practice forgiveness moment by moment, hour by hour, and day by day.

7. **A Test of Commitment:** Keep the promises of God tucked away in your heart. He is trustworthy and loves you. He has a purpose, a plan, a future, and a hope for you. He is making you mature and holy.

8. **A Test of Trust:** Minute by minute surrender all to the Lord.

9. **A Test of Humility:** Become more and more aware of His awesome character. Live a life of meekness and humility as seen in the life of Christ. Christ in us is the hope of glory.

10. **A Test of Dependence:** Commit to living the abundant life in His amazing grace

As we have seen, Scripture records many examples of godly people who have been distracted from goals they have set. In a similar way, the Enemy may attempt to derail your efforts with Thin Within, to distract you from 0 to 5 eating. We encourage you—no matter what trials or tests you endure, no matter how "well" you think you are doing—to keep your focus on the one you serve. Our battle is about so much more than food. It is about the abundant life we have been given in Christ.

Betty, a participant who reached her natural size, said, "I'm no longer afraid to observe what's going on in my life, and I don't judge myself harshly. When I realized weight loss didn't totally hinge on how well I did the program, but was something God was doing in my life, I was able to relax. I recognized that my responsibility is to be in relationship with God and to seek His guidance."

We hope and pray that you will continue, like Betty, to focus on your relationship with God and to seek His guidance. This will be our primary purpose during these last few days.

Take Action

Today we encourage you to renew your commitment to the goals established on Day Three, which were reevaluated on Day Sixteen. These last six days will provide you with an opportunity to give yourself afresh to the Lord. Rely not on your own ability or willpower to accomplish these goals, but instead rely on the grace of God to inspire, equip, and empower you to meet the goals you have set. We encourage you to strengthen or regain your focus and continue forward on the path of His provision.

Lucy, who released over fifty pounds, said, "With Thin Within, you don't need to be perfect, but I came to understand I needed to persevere. Things happen that can seem overwhelming, but now I know how to refocus on God and press on."

We encourage you to rededicate yourself, your praying, your studying, and your energy to accomplishing your goals in the next six days. If Peter could be used of God to bring new life in Christ to three thousand people in one sermon, we know, dear friend, that He can infuse your life with an outpouring of His grace and power in these days remaining before the last page of this book is turned.

Now, let's follow Lucy's example and get refocused.

Thin Within Goal Contract

To assist you in refocusing on your goals, take a look at each goal and break it down into more manageable "action steps."

Begin by asking, "What specific actions must I take to produce goal #1?" Since goal #1 has to do with releasing weight, state these actions with that end specifically in mind. Also, determine when you will take these actions. Space is provided on pages 260–261.

Look at your first goal (Day Sixteen) which had to do with being in a certain dress or pant size by Day Thirty. With six days remaining, what do you think God is leading you to do? Write your adjusted goal under goal #1. Do the same for goals #2 and #3.

Remember, these action steps are designed to assist you in a Spirit-filled walk. Do not allow Larry the Legalist or Abigail the Achiever to convince you to join their ranks. We are called by Christ to run the race with endurance.

The following is an example:

Goal #1. I will release at least two pounds by Day Thirty.

What specific actions do I need to take to produce the results? When will I take these actions?

1. The first action I'll take is to be prayerful.
2. The second action I'll take is to eat 0 to 5 or less for the next six days. I'll choose to let myself feel the 0 for a while before eating.
3. The third action I'll take is to use the Thin Within Keys to Conscious Eating when I choose to eat or drink for the next six days. To help myself, I will copy my Observations and Corrections Chart and use it before and after each meal, or choose some other supportive action.
4. The fourth action I'll take is to move my body in the most enjoyable way for approximately fifteen to thirty minutes each day for the next six days.
5. The fifth action I will take is to spend time with God, asking Him if there is anyone else I need to forgive, and to write forgiveness statements for those people.

Do you get the idea? As with all the other Thin Within exercises, please invite the Spirit of God to direct you. Remember that you have six days left and our God can do amazing things in that time. Be sure you are using your goals from Day Sixteen rather than coming up with new ones.

Date: _____

Goal #1: _____

What specific actions will I take to produce the desired results? When will I take these actions?

1. _____

2. _____

3. _____

4. _____

5. _____

Goal #2: _____

What specific actions will I take to produce the desired results? When will I take these actions?

1. _____

2. _____

3. _____

4. _____

5. _____

Goal #3: _____

What specific actions will I take to produce the desired results? When will I take these actions?

1. _____

2. _____

3. _____

4. _____

5. _____

God's grace has inspired me through His Word. He has equipped me by His Holy Spirit, and I pray that He will continue to empower the results of these action steps, to which I will apply myself for the next six days.

Signed: _____ Date: _____

Weariness may be a part of any journey as worthwhile as the one in which you have been involved. Allow the Lord to renew your strength. As we observed in Isaiah 40, *those who hope in the* LORD *will renew their strength* (emphasis added). Turn to Him, confident of His touch, determined that His grace—pardon, presence, provision, and power—are flowing freely and fully from His throne to you at this very moment.

Let us then approach the throne of grace with confidence, so that we may receive mercy and find grace to help us in our time of need (Hebrews 4:16).

Your Success Story

Record any new insights while you were reading today.

_____

_____

_____

_____

_____

Verses to Ponder

*Consider him who endured such opposition from sinful men, so that you
will not grow weary and lose heart. In your struggle against sin, you have not
yet resisted to the point of shedding your blood* (Hebrews 12:3–4).

*For everything that was written in the past was written to teach us, so that
through endurance and the encouragement of the Scriptures we might have
hope* (Romans 15:4).

*For this reason, since the day we heard about you, we have not stopped pray-
ing for you and asking God to fill you with the knowledge of his will through
all spiritual wisdom and understanding. And we pray this in order that you
may live a life worthy of the Lord and may please him in every way: bearing
fruit in every good work, growing in the knowledge of God, being strengthened
with all power according to his glorious might so that you may have great
endurance and patience, and joyfully giving thanks to the Father, who has
qualified you to share in the inheritance of the saints in the kingdom of light.
For he has rescued us from the dominion of darkness and brought us into the
kingdom of the Son he loves, in whom we have redemption, the forgiveness of
sins* (Colossians 1:9–14).

Prayer

*Lord, thank You that Your grace gives me the inspiration and strength to
endure. Help me to persevere toward the goals You have set before me. I
pray I will not abuse Your grace, Lord, but will allow it to mature me.
Give me patience to wait on You to feed me with the choicest of foods and
help me, Lord, to cling to You as I walk in the truth of who I am in Christ.
Help me surrender my will as I cling tenaciously to You. In Christ's
name, Amen.*

Success Tools

+ Fill in the Hunger Graph.
+ Fill in the Thin Within Food Log.
+ Mark the Thin Within Observations and Corrections Chart for today.
+ Use the Thin Within Keys to Conscious Eating.
+ Use the Gratitude List or your Thanksgiving Journal to record what
  you are thankful for.

Medical Moment

We are told in Genesis that life will be difficult, and the history of humankind documents this fact. Trials and stress have always been with us and seem to be increasing with time. The question of what effect this has on our health has long been a concern. When we are stressed, increased amounts of adrenaline and cortisol are secreted by our adrenal glands. As a result, blood pressure and heart rate increase while blood is selectively diverted from the intestinal tract to the brain and extremity muscles for a "fight or flight" response.

When the stress is relieved, secretion of these hormones is reduced and the body returns to its "resting" state. But what is the effect of persistent stress? Chronically elevated levels of adrenaline and cortisol can contribute to hypertension, heart disease, stroke, and a variety of intestinal problems including peptic ulcer disease and irritable bowel syndrome, suppression of the immune system, headaches, insomnia, possible sexual dysfunction, and a host of psychiatric problems. What is the answer to chronic stress? In a word, it is to rest in the Lord—to know that He is in charge, that our past is forgiven, the Holy Spirit is with us in the present, and our future is secured. *Do not be wise in your own eyes; fear the LORD and shun evil. This will bring health to your body and nourishment to your bones* (Proverbs 3:7–8).

—Arthur Halliday, M.D.

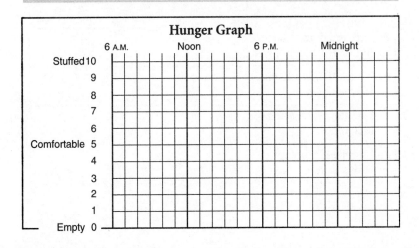

Hunger Graph

Thin Within Food Log

Hunger # before Eating	Time	Items/Amount	Hunger # after Eating

Thin Within Observations and Corrections Chart—Day 24

Observations	Day 24
1. I ate when my body was hungry.	
2. I ate in a calm environment by reducing distractions.	
3. I ate when I was sitting.	
4. I ate when my body and mind were relaxed.	
5. I ate and drank the things my body enjoyed.	
6. I paid attention to my food while eating.	
7. I ate slowly, savoring each bite.	
8. I stopped before my body was full.	

Gratitude List

_____

_____

_____

Thin Within Wisdom

Keep your eyes on Him. He alone is faithful.

Broadening Godly Boundaries

The day for building your walls will come,
the day for extending your boundaries.
—Micah 7:11

A celebration is imminent! The day is coming when you will commemorate the completion of your restoration project. Soon the work will be done. It stands before us now, an accolade of the grace of God winding as a banner of victory through our lives.

We have cooperated with our God to build upon His foundation of truth, set with sturdy pylons of grace to the bedrock of Christ. Before we halt the mallet and chisel, before we allow ourselves the privilege of resting in the shade, let's complete the tasks at hand. The day has come for us to be sure that the wall is firmly set and the boundary stones placed according to God's direction. Let's reaffirm that our city walls are fortified and that the temple that resides within is secure from enemy assault.

During Day Eighteen we established some godly boundaries. We spoke of Nehemiah, who established and maintained his personal boundaries while respecting the boundaries of God.

As you refocus during these last five days on the goals set before you, seeking to win the prize of the abundant holy life, you may have overlooked some possible distractions that can come from within your "walls." Family and friends, perhaps unintentionally, can be one of the primary vehicles through which we are tempted to abandon our boundaries. Those we live with at home and those we spend time with at work, church, school, or in our community can very easily tempt us away from conscious eating.

Have you already noticed this possible pitfall?

Let's start with your immediate family. By now you have identified your "whole-body pleasers" and have established your personal boundaries regarding what and when you will eat. Believing that your body is trustworthy and capable of telling you what it needs no longer seems like an unrealistic idea.

If you have involved others in eating the Thin Within way, you have undoubtedly learned that others have different pleasers and teasers than you do. That doesn't have to spell disaster. In fact it can be a chance to broaden your own food boundaries. You may end up discovering some new and exciting pleasers that you've never tried before. You can also inspire your family members to make similar discoveries.

Today let's consider occasions that involve eating with others.

Take Action

Eating the Thin Within Way with My Family Exercise

Think of a typical meal with your family. What obstacles may prevent you or your family from following the keys to conscious eating? Record these in the left-hand column. Don't write the solutions quite yet.

Potential Obstacles	Creative Solutions
Every child has a different pleaser.	
My husband comes home and wants to eat and I'm not at a 0 yet.	

In the activity on page 268 we have identified five common purposes for eating at home. Feel free to add to that list any purposes you have for eating with your children, husband, roommate.

My Purpose in Eating at Home
1. Satisfying hunger
2. Conversation
3. Convenience
4. Together time
5. Learning proper table etiquette
6._____
7._____
8._____
9._____
10._____

Determining your main purposes when eating with others will help you find solutions to the obstacles you listed on page 267. If you know what your primary purpose is, you can focus on that instead of eating. For instance, when Don and Carol realized they could sit and talk with their young children at the dinner table without feeling compelled to eat with them, their relationship with the children vastly improved.

Speaking of children, they can be good examples of those who trust their bodies and are naturally thin eaters. You might be concerned about your children getting all the nutrients they need, especially if their eating habits seem to you to be bizarre. However, children are generally able to hear and respond to the signals of their God-given bodies. Over the years a number of experiments have validated that if children are allowed to choose without restrictions from a wide variety of foods, they will generally choose only sweets for the first few days, after which they will start making wiser food choices. They'll discover that sweets in excess aren't whole-body pleasers and will eventually choose a healthier selection of foods. Observe your child for a couple of weeks and see what happens. Remember the importance of providing a selection of nutritious foods.

Knowing that children will instinctively eat nutritiously if allowed to choose from a variety of healthy foods means parents no longer need to nag at their kids about what they do or don't eat. When they have the freedom to choose from what is offered, and the parents can give them their undivided attention, the eating experience will be much more pleasant and meaningful for everyone.

Perhaps you have a family where no two people have the same "pleasers." A suggestion to consider when planning ahead is to allow each person, including the kids, to pick their pleaser for an evening meal. This will be fun and it will also relieve the one who usually cooks the meals from having to be creative every day.

At the Anderson home the family planned the evening meals for the week in advance. Each person picked one day and was then allowed to choose the pleaser for that evening's meal. This was recorded on the weekly menu and the necessary ingredients were written on the shopping list. The meal-planning experience even solved some mealtime problems as all agreed to participate in the plan without grumbling. It was an enjoyable project, the kids loved it, and the family gained a sense of teamwork.

Whenever you feel yourself hindered from following the keys to conscious eating, seek God's grace and wisdom in determining a solution. As you maintain godly boundaries within your family setting, your children will be less likely to have problems related to eating when they are older. Now return to the exercise on page 267 called Eating the Thin Within Way with My Family and record your "creative solutions."

Eating the Thin Within Way with Friends and Extended Family

Now consider a large family gathering, a church potluck, a business lunch, or a birthday party. Write down any situations that might make it difficult to apply the keys to conscious eating. By planning ahead to maintain your boundaries in a social setting, you can take a proactive approach. You can *respond*, rather than *react* if you plan in advance.

For instance, if there are many different types of food from which to choose, that may increase the likelihood of more whole-body pleasers, which will make your 0 to 5 eating experience easier and more enjoyable. Be very selective, eating only those things that you really know are whole-body pleasers. If you think there may be only a few pleasers from which to choose, you may want to eat a pleaser at home and arrive at the occasion at a 3 on the hunger scale. Then you won't have to eat much to reach your comfortable 5.

Ask the Lord how you can take these potential stumbling blocks and turn them into building stones for the restoration and maintenance of your godly temple.

With that in mind, fill in the following chart.

Potluck

Potential Obstacles	Creative Solutions
Abundance of food.	
Too many varieties to choose from.	
Worry about what people will think of me if I eat too little or too much.	

Denise describes one way she has learned to handle the challenge of eating with a group: "Now, if I don't want to miss the occasion but also I don't want to eat, I just have something to drink. People don't usually notice or care whether or not you eat."

It may be helpful to take a personal inventory prior to attending a social occasion. Pray for wisdom, then ask yourself, "Why am I going to this particular event and what do I hope to gain from it?" It's doubtful that your answer will be "I want to overeat." Planning ahead will help you to honor your godly boundaries and avoid situations that lead to inappropriate eating. You may conclude that you really do want to go to some events but that eating is your last priority. Or you may decide that you would prefer doing something else instead. Remember it's OK to say "no."

However, if you choose to go to a social event that includes food and eating, it will be very helpful to define your purpose in attending this event.

My Purpose in Going to This Social Occasion
1. Make new acquaintances
2. Fun
3. Business contacts
4. Eat the food because the chef is excellent.
5. _____
6. _____
7. _____
8. _____

Eating at a restaurant doesn't have to derail your efforts to maintain your godly boundaries. When Arthur and I eat out, we often order two salads, one entrée, one dessert, and we may still have leftovers. This really reduces the expense of eating out and makes our dining experience quite enjoyable. Portions served these days are huge, and there's no need to allow our culture with its mega-sizes to dictate how much we eat.

Rhonda and her family share meals out with their seven-year-old daughter. The child, rather than being limited to a children's menu, is able to taste a broad variety of foods. The family saves money and no one overeats. Since the waiter or waitress brings them an extra plate and accommodates their requests, they leave a generous tip expressing their appreciation.

Denise has a very creative solution. "When I eat out," she shares, "I take a disposable takeout container with me because it's difficult to get a waiter to bring a container along with the food. This may sound like a rude thing to do. However, I know if there's food on the plate in front of me, I'll eat it. So when the meal arrives, whatever I am not planning to eat goes into the container which I take home to eat at another time." One participant reports that she was served so much food during a single Mexican dinner that she took home enough leftovers for four more adequately portioned meals!

If you remain committed to your goals, with your boundaries firmly fixed, eating wisely will become second nature and will require less energy with time. You will want to remain vigilant, however, to sustain the success you have enjoyed this far. And rest assured that you can ask God to set off a "Holy Spirit alarm" when a potential encroachment to your boundaries draws near. Trust Him. Listen to Him. Obey His voice.

Devote yourselves to prayer, being watchful and thankful (Colossians 4:2).

Your Success Story
Record any new insights while you were reading today.

Verses to Ponder

They will celebrate your abundant goodness and joyfully sing of your righteousness (Psalm 145:7).

They will come and shout for joy on the heights of Zion; they will rejoice in the bounty of the LORD—the grain, the new wine and the oil, the young of the flocks and herds. They will be like a well-watered garden, and they will sorrow no more. Then maidens will dance and be glad, young men and old as well. I will turn their mourning into gladness; I will give them comfort and joy instead of sorrow. I will satisfy the priests with abundance, and my people will be filled with my bounty," declares the LORD (Jeremiah 31:12–14).

The jailer brought them into his house and set a meal before them; he was filled with joy because he had come to believe in God—he and his whole family (Acts 16:34).

Prayer

Lord, please help me to extend, establish, and maintain godly boundaries where my food choices and relationships are concerned. I want to continue with 0 to 5 eating, and I don't want to use social occasions as an excuse to eat according to my "flesh machinery." Lord, I know that at all times I need to lean on You, because it is by Your grace alone that I can continue to stand firm, eating only when I am hungry and stopping when I am comfortable. Thank You for the confidence I can have in You, Lord. When I am weak, You are strong. In Jesus' name, Amen.

Medical Moment

As we have previously said, our prayer for each of you is that you will experience physical, emotional, and spiritual health. This, of course, is never one hundred percent attainable as we all fall short of the glory of God. But there are many things we can do that will enhance all aspects of our health. There is a burgeoning field in medicine called "psychoneuroimmunology," which deals with the relationship between our emotions and our susceptibility to disease, our overall health, and even how long we live. It has been established that there is a direct correlation, either positive or negative, between the state of our mind and our health. Good relationships, rewarding jobs, harmonious families, a feeling of being valued, worthwhile community or church service, a sense that we are fulfilling God's plan for our lives, all can contribute to a more meaningful and much healthier life. With the Lord's help, shift your attention away from a preoccupation with food and eating. The payoff is that you will have more energy that can be directed toward the goal of faithful service for God.

—ARTHUR HALLIDAY, M.D.

Success Tools

+ Fill in the Hunger Graph.
+ Fill in the Thin Within Food Log.
+ Use the Thin Within Observations and Corrections Chart for today.
+ Use the Thin Within Keys to Conscious Eating.
+ Use the Gratitude List or your Thanksgiving Journal to record your blessings.

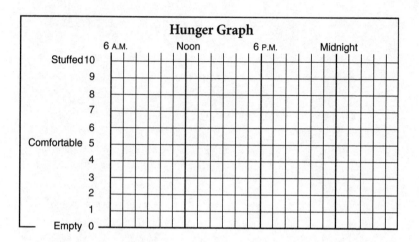

Thin Within Food Log

Hunger # before Eating	Time	Items/Amount	Hunger # after Eating

Thin Within Observations and Corrections Chart—Day 25

Observations	Day 25
1. I ate when my body was hungry.	
2. I ate in a calm environment by reducing distractions.	
3. I ate when I was sitting.	
4. I ate when my body and mind were relaxed.	
5. I ate and drank the things my body enjoyed.	
6. I paid attention to my food while eating.	
7. I ate slowly, savoring each bite.	
8. I stopped before my body was full.	

Gratitude List

_____

_____

_____

Thin Within Wisdom

Maintain godly boundaries even when enjoying a social occasion to help you reach and maintain your God-given natural size.

The Adventure of His Abundance

O God, you are my God, earnestly I seek you;
my soul thirsts for you, my body longs for you,
in a dry and weary land where there is no water.
I have seen you in the sanctuary
and beheld your power and your glory.
Because your love is better than life,
my lips will glorify you.
I will praise you as long as I live,
and in your name I will lift up my hands.
My soul will be satisfied as with the richest of foods.
With singing lips my mouth will praise you.
—Psalm 63:1–5

Have you ever felt this sort of yearning that the psalmist speaks about? Over the past twenty-five days we have sought to tap into the vast resources of God to satisfy our longings. He is a fountain of living water that knows no measure. The depth of His love is deeper than the deepest sea. His bounty is so immense that just to taste of it is to fall to our knees in awe and worship.

The LORD will guide you always; he will satisfy your needs in a sun-scorched land and will strengthen your frame. You will be like a well-watered garden, like a spring whose waters never fail (Isaiah 58:11).

The Lord alone can satisfy the emptiness in our souls and the needs for which our hearts yearn. It is a refrain that we've been singing since the onset of our journey, and it is the victory song that we'll sing for eternity. Christ is sufficient. He is more than enough.

For in Christ all the fullness of the Deity lives in bodily form, and you have been given fullness in Christ . . . (Colossians 2:9–10a).

Yes, we have been given fullness in Christ. But if we are honest, many of us would have to admit that there still seems to be something missing. There is a tendency of our flesh to insist on chasing after something else, some missing piece, to satisfy our insatiable thirst for love and acceptance.

We still may find ourselves tempted to run from one thing to another, hoping to stifle our inner yearnings with counterfeits. As A. W. Tozer writes, "I want deliberately to encourage this mighty longing after God. He waits to be wanted. Too bad that with many of us He waits so long, so very long, in vain. The simplicity, which is in Christ, is rarely found among us. In its stead are programs, methods, organizations and a world of nervous activities, which occupy time and attention but can never satisfy the longing of the heart."[1]

As Tozer points out, there is a need for us to distinguish between the "real thing" and the counterfeits of life. As we have discovered in our experiences with food and our bodies, more is *not* better. In the past we may have thought so, but what we try to stuff into the void isn't what the void was designed to carry. Food, clothes, cars, accomplishments, performance, sex, titles, awards, or approval from others can't fill a void that was created only for God. The results of our efforts will at best be disappointing and, at the worst, devastating.

King Solomon tried to fill the longings of his heart with anything and everything but God. In the book of Ecclesiastes, which many believe was authored by Solomon, he recounts his efforts to give his life meaning. Wisdom alone didn't do it. Wine, women, and song didn't do it. Building bigger and better houses, parks, wonders of the world didn't do it. Amassing gold, silver, and great wealth didn't satisfy him.

I denied myself nothing my eyes desired; I refused my heart no pleasure. My heart took delight in all my work, and this was the reward for all my labor. Yet when I surveyed all that my hands had done and what I had toiled to achieve, everything was meaningless, a chasing after the wind; nothing was gained under the sun (Ecclesiastes 2:10–11).

After all this, Solomon described his conclusion, *Meaningless. It was all meaningless. It was a chasing after the wind. Nothing was gained.* He was so right. Trying to satisfy our God-given heart hunger with things of this world, with anything other than God is meaningless.

Over the past twenty-six days you've learned not to expect food to satisfy anything but an empty stomach. Have you found yourself drawn to something else as you've tried to quiet the cravings of your soul? Now that you are putting food in its proper place, has it been replaced by anything in your life other than the Lord?

For instance, have you found yourself spending more money? If you once thought, "more food is better" are you now acting as if "more is better" in recreational pursuits? Knowledge? Work? Movies or books? It is entirely possible to satisfactorily resolve issues of food and eating and still not turn to our Lord to satisfy the hunger of our hearts.

Let's take a moment to contemplate and compare satisfaction and gratification.

Satisfaction: This word can be applied to a heart that has been sustained or a need that has been fulfilled by God's provision. When the need no longer cries out to be met and another does not rise up in its place, we are satisfied. When our bodies call out for food, we have learned that this physical hunger can be satisfied with a small, fist-sized amount of food. Eating what God provides when our body needs it will leave us physically satisfied. Better still, our soul or heart hunger will be satisfied by constant fellowship with our Creator.

Gratification: This word describes temporary or immediate pleasure. It may be the candy bar that you thought would "feed a need." When you finished, the burst of joy it gave you was only temporary. Even when we are physically hungry, food can't satisfy the needs of our hearts. There is something else that still cries out for satisfaction.

Satisfaction and gratification can perhaps best be compared side by side.

Figure 26-1 on page 280 illustrates the path of my performance, which is a life of temporary gratification, and the path of God's provision, which is a life of sustained satisfaction as we find ourselves continuing to turn to God.

We can remain in a place of heart and soul satisfaction when we surrender our will, mind, emotions, unmet needs, and our bodies to our Heavenly Father. Remaining on the path of God's provision will allow for this blessing to be ours! Isaiah declares:

Come, all you who are thirsty, come to the waters; and you, who have no money, come, buy and eat! Come, buy wine and milk without money and without cost. Why spend money on what is not bread, and your labor on what does not satisfy? Listen, listen to me, and eat what is good, and your soul will delight in the richest of fare. Give ear and come to me; hear me that your soul may live. I will make an everlasting covenant with you, my faithful love promised to David (Isaiah 55:1–3).

Our soul experiences satisfaction as we reflectively abide in Him and are willing to be made mature. In seeking satisfaction we develop patience and perseverance. We wait for our 0 with a knowledge that the spirit within will have the final word.

Gratification, on the other hand, is always temporary. We have learned in past weeks how God has designed us so that we can distinguish between the hunger of the heart, which no worldly thing can satisfy, and the legitimate physiological hunger that occurs when our body requires nourishment. Discerning between the two and seeking appropriate satisfaction is one of our primary goals.

Satisfaction	Gratification
1. Comes from within. It is a state of the heart that is at peace with our Maker. God's ample provision puts an end to a need and provides sustained heart and soul satisfaction.	1. Comes from outside of ourselves. Anything that we seek to satisfy our hungry hearts, that affords only temporary pleasure. The need remains. (Romans 13:14; Galatians 5:16)
2. Comes from a personal relationship with a risen Christ and a correct view of ourselves through God's eyes. a. My body is the temple of the Holy Spirit. I am not my own. I was bought at a price. (1 Corinthians 6:19–20) b. Keeping our commitments by the grace of God at work within me. (Numbers 30:2) c. Doing the best job we can do. (1 Corinthians 10:31) d. Be willing to surrender our will and rights. (Philippians 3:2–8) e. Pressing beyond our comfort zone. Allowing God to use us for His purposes. (Romans 9:20–21)	2. Comes from a temporary or immediate pleasure. (2 Timothy 2:2–7) a. Movies b. Manicure c. Food/drink d. TV e. Spectator sports f. Shopping g. Etc.
3. Earned by Christ and given to us through Him. (Colossians 2:9–10)	3. Not earned. (Ephesians 2:3)

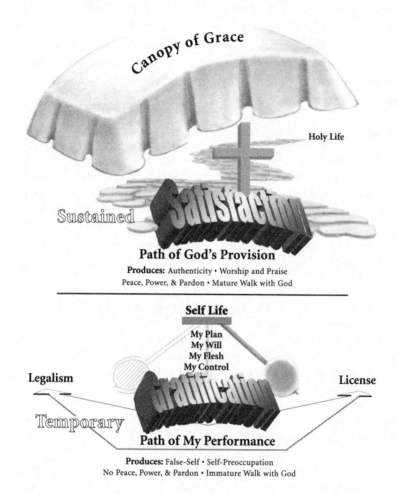

Canopy of Grace

Holy Life

Sustained **Satisfaction**

Path of God's Provision

Produces: Authenticity • Worship and Praise
Peace, Power, & Pardon • Mature Walk with God

Self Life

My Plan
My Will
My Flesh
My Control

Legalism   License

Temporary **Gratification**

Path of My Performance

Produces: False-Self • Self-Preoccupation
No Peace, Power, & Pardon • Immature Walk with God

figure 26–1

Tammy, who has released over two hundred pounds to date, says, "For me, overeating resulted from not having an intimate relationship with God. Before Thin Within I believed in God, but I didn't know what an intimate relationship with Him was." She discovered that the longings of her heart, which she had previously attempted to feed with food, were actually longings for the Lord. Food never satisfied her heart hunger, but she continued to eat, not knowing what else to do. Once she began to feed her hungry heart with an intimacy that comes only from the Lord, she experienced real satisfaction, and her overeating was halted. We are hopeful that you, too, have begun to turn to the Lord, asking Him to fill the deep longing that only He can satisfy.

Take Action

The following exercise has been extremely beneficial to many Thin Within participants and is designed to help you turn away from the counterfeit forms of satisfaction. We offer an example in this "good-bye to food" letter.

Dear Food,

Writing to you has been in my mind and on my heart for a very long time. I know you may not be expecting this, and that it may even be a shock to you, but I may as well say it directly. Food, I need to break up with you. You see, I have discovered that I turned to you to satisfy what only Another can satisfy. You have been a great disappointment and have not given me what I've needed. You promised me that you would always be there to meet all of the needs of my heart, but I have found your promises to be empty. Sure, we have had some good times together—on vacation, watching movies, at parties and potlucks, but I made you more important than people and much more important than God. It isn't fair or right for me to continue depending on you to deliver something that you just can't supply.

I expected so many things of you. I thought you would make me happy but you haven't. The truth is I have been miserable. I thought that you would make my pain go away, but you didn't. I thought you would fill the emptiness, but you couldn't. In fact, I also blamed you for many of my problems. I now see that I must take responsibility for those things and take them to the only one who can satisfy me with His truth and His life. We will always be together and can still be friends, but you can no longer be my best friend or secret love. I can no longer live for you, but I will come to you for the only thing you are able to give me—physical nourishment.

> *Sincerely,*
> *(your name)*

The Book of Ecclesiastes is, in essence, King Solomon's "good-bye letter to everything else." It ends with this:

Now all has been heard; here is the conclusion of the matter: Fear God and keep his commandments, for this is the whole duty of man (Ecclesiastes 12:13).

You may be uncertain as to Solomon's conclusion, wondering why "fearing God" is something that could reflect a life of satisfaction. What does it mean to "fear God?" A biblical fear of the Lord is an awe that calls us to authentic worship. It is a healthy, accurate view of God that sees the Lord as He is, high and exalted, and ourselves as humble and dependent. When we cease relating to God as our "buddy," as a God of convenience, and when we esteem Him in His rightful place of honor, we humbly surrender ourselves and our choices to Him. We no longer view His grace simply as "a terrific deal" to cover all our sin (which it does), but we see it as a power that sustains our obedient choices, causing us to will and to do according to His good pleasure. This mature walk with the Lord refuses to diminish the awesomeness of God, but allows Him to be Lord in all ways, with tenderness and compassion, justice, holiness, and truth. This is the true biblical fear of God. *The fear of the* LORD *is the beginning of wisdom* (Proverbs 9:10).

Solomon declared that by developing a fear or reverence of the Lord, he was able to say good-bye to all of those things which could not begin to satisfy the emptiness in his heart.

Perhaps you don't need to write a "good-bye to food" letter. However, there may be something else you have misused in a similar way, trying to fill that hunger in your heart with some other counterfeit. Take time to prayerfully consider what it is you need to "release" or surrender to the Lord. If you turn to anything other than God for heart and soul satisfaction, it is time for you to "break up."

Good-bye to _____ Letter

Date: _____

Dear _____,

_____

_____

_____

Signed _____

D. L. Moody has said, "The world cannot satisfy our new nature [new man]. No earthly well can satisfy the soul, which has become a partaker of the heavenly nature.

Honor, wealth, and the pleasures of this world, will not satisfy those who, having gone astray, are again earnestly searching for the living water.

Earthly wells will get dry—by-and-by, if not now; and they will not quench spiritual thirst."[2]

Do you dare to relinquish, to surrender anything that remains firmly in your grip? We pray that you will and in turn you will be filled to overflowing with His peace, joy, and enduring satisfaction.

Your Success Story

Did you have any new insights while you were reading today? Please record them below.

_____

_____

_____

_____

Verses to Ponder

But you would be fed with the finest of wheat; with honey from the rock I would satisfy you (Psalm 81:16).

Praise the LORD, O my soul, and forget not all his benefits . . . who satisfies your desires with good things so that your youth is renewed like the eagle's (Psalm 103:2, 5).

Let them give thanks to the LORD for his unfailing love and his wonderful deeds for men, for he satisfies the thirsty and fills the hungry with good things (Psalm 107:8–9).

Prayer

Dear Lord, forgive me for the times that I have turned to food to try and satisfy my deeper longing for You. I know that nothing can quench the thirst of my soul but You. Thank You for teaching me the proper place food is to have in my life. Help me now to see and to release to You any worldly dependencies that I cling to, and to trust You as You teach me about making mature and excellent choices that require wisdom and patience. I pray that I might be wholly surrendered and given over to You. In Jesus' name, Amen.

Medical Moment

As theologians ask "how then shall we live?" gerontologists ask "how long shall we then live?"—a question complicated by concerns we all have about the infirmities to which we are subject as we age. The idealized scenario of some is that we would remain healthy until age 120 and then die peacefully in our sleep. The following list is adapted from the Tufts University Health letter of April 2001, to which we would add a strong belief and faith in our Almighty God who loves each and every one of us.

1. Sleep seven to eight hours per night.
2. Maintain optimum weight.
3. Exercise thirty minutes daily.
4. Avoid alcohol or limit consumption—to no more than one drink daily for women, or two for men.
5. Avoid tobacco.
6. Eat breakfast when you reach your 0.
7. Avoid frequent snacking.
8. Never quit learning.
9. Stay socially connected.
10. Maintain optimism.

Long life to you! Good health to you and your household! And
good health to all that is yours!
—1 Samuel 25:6

—ARTHUR HALLIDAY, M.D.

Success Tools

+ Fill in the Hunger Graph.
+ Fill in the Thin Within Food Log.
+ Use the Thin Within Observations and Corrections Chart for today.
+ Use the Thin Within Keys to Conscious Eating.
+ Use the Gratitude List or your Thanksgiving Journal to record your blessings.

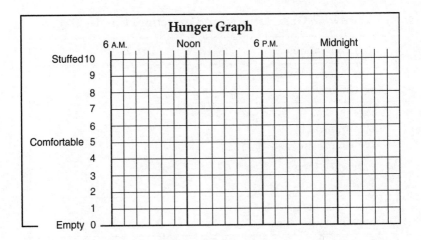

Thin Within Food Log

Hunger # before Eating	Time	Items/Amount	Hunger # after Eating

Gratitude List

_____

_____

_____

Thin Within Wisdom

Dare to relinquish or surrender anything that remains firmly in your grip.

Thin Within Observations and Corrections Chart—Day 26

Observations	Day 26
1. I ate when my body was hungry.	
2. I ate in a calm environment by reducing distractions.	
3. I ate when I was sitting.	
4. I ate when my body and mind were relaxed.	
5. I ate and drank the things my body enjoyed.	
6. I paid attention to my food while eating.	
7. I ate slowly, savoring each bite.	
8. I stopped before my body was full.	

NOTES
1. A. W. Tozer, *The Pursuit of God* (Camp Hill, Pennsylvania: Christian Publications, Inc., 1982), 17.
2. D. L. Moody.

Complete in His Tenderness: Part 1

Turn my eyes away from worthless things;
preserve my life according to your word.
—Psalm 119:37

Your temple stands almost complete, only a few finishing touches remain. With God's help you have diligently rebuilt, fortified, and restored His dwelling place. Soon you will have the privilege of maintaining it. You have turned your eyes away from worthless things and fixed them upon the Lord who loves you. You have obeyed his call.

"Come to me, all you who are weary and burdened, and I will give you rest" (Matthew 11:28).

He says, "Come to me. If you are weary, if you are burdened. Come, come to me. I will give you . . ."

". . . More burdens to carry?"

No. Mercifully not.

". . . More rules to follow?"

No. Grace abounds instead.

". . . More people to please?"

No. We seek to please only our God.

I will give you rest . . .

Do you hear it? Jesus knows when we are weary and burdened. He will give us rest if we will but come to Him (Matthew 11:28). When we are weary, we are vulnerable—vulnerable to flesh-filled eating, vulnerable to focusing on performance instead of God's provision, and vulnerable to turning to temporary gratification rather than to the true life-sustaining satisfaction found only in Him.

Why Weariness?

There are several reasons why we may grow weary. And by "weary," we don't simply mean physically tiredness. We mean that beaten-down, hard-to-get-out-of, can't-take-much-more sort of feeling. We're talking about mental and spiritual as well as physical exhaustion, when life has become a list of "must dos" instead of an adventure blessed with wonder, joy, and abundance. This is the kind of weariness that tarnishes the soul's luster.

So what causes us to feel weary? We are going to focus on three reasons. To do this, however, take an honest look at your schedule for the upcoming week and use the calendar below to record your activities.

Start with the first thing you have planned to do tomorrow and fill in the appropriate space. Please don't forget to include time for reading your Bible as well as for reading *Thin Within*.

	Sunday	Monday	Tuesday	Wednesday	Thursday	Friday	Saturday
6 A.M.							
7 A.M.							
8 A.M.							
9 A.M.							
10 A.M.							
11 A.M.							
Noon							
1 P.M.							
2 P.M.							
3 P.M.							
4 P.M.							
5 P.M.							
6 P.M.							
7 P.M.							
8 P.M.							
9 P.M.							

Now review your schedule and see if you need to add anything, such as time you spend driving to and from work, school, or appointments.

People generally become weary for one of three reasons:[1]

Reason #1: We invest ourselves in things that are not part of God's plan.

Have you ever asked God about your schedule? If not, consider doing so. Our time is the most valuable thing we have, and He cares about each and every detail of our lives. Are there activities or responsibilities that God perhaps has been calling you to surrender to Him, even things that might be categorized as "socially acceptable?" Do you hear His kind voice telling you to follow Him, away from that extra social event, late-night TV show, extra bridge class, sixty-hour work week, surfing the Internet at work? How many self-improvement books does He really want you to read? How many of these activities would you let go of if Jesus were physically present with you? (He is, in fact!)

Look over your schedule for the upcoming week and pray that God will show you what falls outside His plan for you. Put a colored mark next to each item that you think may be something God is calling you to release.

I desire to do your will, O my God; your law is within my heart (Psalms 40:8).

Reason #2: We invest ourselves in godly activities beyond God's plan.

Finding unnecessary godly activities on your schedule may be a bit tricky because they are "good" things. But is it really His plan for you to attend yet another fellowship group? Or perhaps you said "yes" when the ministry coordinator at your church asked you to take on an additional Bible study because no one else was available. Have you taken on too much all in the name of godly service? Is it possible that you are not adhering to godly boundaries? Prayerfully look again at your schedule. Use a *different* mark for any of those things in your schedule that may represent going beyond what God has called you to do.

Paul effectively stated the solution to this dilemma of having so many "good" things in his life.

But whatever was to my profit I now consider loss for the sake of Christ. What is more, I consider everything a loss compared to the surpassing greatness of knowing Christ Jesus my Lord, for whose sake I have lost all things. I consider them rubbish, that I may gain Christ (Philippians 3:7–8).

Paul wanted only God's best. The same standard should apply to us. Even "good" things that God has called you to do must be counted as loss compared to your intimate fellowship with Him and your heart seeking after Christ.

It is helpful to remember that sometimes Jesus left places in which He ministered before He had healed all the people waiting to see Him, before all who needed Him had been touched. Yet at the end of His earthly life, *Jesus prayed to the Father, "I have brought you glory on earth by completing the work you gave me to do"* (John 17:4). Some were still sick. Some were still blind. But Jesus had done all He was called to do.

There will be times when we disappoint people by saying "no." There will always be a need for another nursery worker, another PTA volunteer, another choir member, another car-pool driver. While you can remain compassionate, prayerful, and ready to serve, always listen carefully for God's leading, refusing to be led into weariness by responding to the wrong voices. Remember, His voice is the one that says, clearly, "Come . . . come . . . I will give you rest . . ." Heeding His voice is not only "good" but "excellent" in His eyes!

Reason #3: We rely on our own strength rather than God's in doing what He's called us to do.

Even those things that God calls us to do, when done in our own strength, can be exhausting. By contrast, if you are energized in your spirit by doing it, chances are you are doing it in His strength.

At the present time, are there godly things you are doing in your own strength? How could you begin to do them in His strength? Write your thoughts and observations here.

_____

_____

_____

Some people believe the "work of God" should be joyless drudgery. How can that be? With Christ as our example, we quickly see that nothing could be further from the truth. A life lived in the power of the Spirit, as illustrated in Day Four, is an abundant holy life. Life in Him is not free of challenges, but it exudes joy and peace. Jesus knew how to enjoy life and He has called us to go in and out as we enjoy safe pastures (John 10:9b).

Prayerfully invite God to reveal those things in your upcoming schedule that you are called to do relying on His strength. Now please *rewrite* your schedule. Leave out anything that is outside of God's plan for you—those things you identified in reason #1 and #2 with marks next to them.

	Sunday	Monday	Tuesday	Wednesday	Thursday	Friday	Saturday
6 A.M.							
7 A.M.							
8 A.M.							
9 A.M.							
10 A.M.							
11 A.M.							
Noon							
1 P.M.							
2 P.M.							
3 P.M.							
4 P.M.							
5 P.M.							
6 P.M.							
7 P.M.							
8 P.M.							
9 P.M.							

Whatever God has truly called you to do, you can do in His strength, and He will give you His peace and His joy in the process. If He calls you, He equips you. Jesus doesn't want you to be weary and burdened down. You are His precious sheep, the one that He has sought to lead and nurture. You are His lamb to whom he said . . .

"This is the resting place, let the weary rest"; and, "This is the place of repose"—but they would not listen. So then, the word of the LORD to them will become: Do and do, do and do, rule on rule, rule on rule; a little here, a little

there—so that they will go and fall backward, be injured and snared and cap-tured (Isaiah 28:12–13).

Our Lord has spoken to us. We've heard His voice. He wants you to come to Him, to let go of your burden and the weariness it has caused. On the path of God's provision, He says, "This is the resting place, let the weary rest."

Take Action

Look at the things in your first schedule that aren't listed on your second schedule. (All of those things with your two marks on them.) Can you make these changes a reality in the week ahead? Can you make phone calls and cancel appointments? Can you apologize if necessary and recruit others to take on a task? We hope the idea of making changes in your schedule restores your hope and gives you joy.

Come to me, all you who are weary and burdened, and I will give you rest. Take my yoke upon you and learn from me, for I am gentle and humble in heart, and you will find rest for your souls. For my yoke is easy and my burden is light (Matthew 11:28–30).

Tomorrow you will look again at your "new" schedule and the yoke to which Jesus calls you to submit. As you consider your schedule for the next three days, remember to include your time in the Bible and *Thin Within*. Tomorrow we will focus on an additional reason that we may experience weariness. We will investigate what happens when we, like Jonah, hear the call of God and refuse to obey. Our Lord wants us to experience his rest, His gentleness, His humble heart, His ease, and His light load. And by God's grace we will.

Your Success Story

Did you have any new insights while you were reading today? Please record them below.

_____

_____

_____

Verses to Ponder

Remain in me, and I will remain in you. No branch can bear fruit by itself; it must remain in the vine. Neither can you bear fruit unless you remain in me (John 15:4).

. . . His incomparably great power [is] for us who believe. That power is like the working of his mighty strength, which he exerted in Christ when he raised him from the dead and seated him at his right hand in the heavenly realms (Ephesians 1:19–20).

I can do everything through him who gives me strength (Philippians 4:13).

Prayer

Lord, it is so hard to say "no." So many demands are made on my time, and I know that when my life becomes fragmented I am far more vulnerable to following flesh-filled eating. Lord, I've come so far and I want to continue to focus on You and the satisfaction and rest that only You can give. Help me to have the courage and strength to make changes in my schedule that will reflect a life that is directed and empowered only by Your Holy Spirit. In Jesus' name, Amen.

Medical Moment

The industrial revolution that burst on to the scene in England 150 years ago was widely seen to herald man's triumph over nature. It was believed that machines would raise the standard of living for the millions of underprivileged around the world. The record of science since then and continuing today has seen a succession of technological advances beyond our wildest dreams, but which at times appears to proceed almost out of control. Sadly it seems that the pace and quality of life, rather than improving, has further polarized the haves and the have nots, at times threatening planet earth and perhaps the entire human race. Caught up in the frantic pace of modern life, we are losing our capacity for inner contemplation. The only answer is to return to our Creator, acknowledging that His ways, not ours, are the only hope to save humanity from itself.

Praise the LORD, O my soul, and forget not all His benefits—who forgives all your sins and heals all your diseases, who redeems your life from the pit and crowns you with love and compassion, who satisfies your desires with good things so that your youth is renewed like the eagle's.
—Psalm 103:2–5

—ARTHUR HALLIDAY, M.D.

Success Tools

✦ Fill in the Hunger Graph.

✦ Fill in the Thin Within Food Log.

✦ Use the Thin Within Observations and Corrections Chart for today.

✦ Use the Thin Within Keys to Conscious Eating.

✦ Use the Gratitude List or your Thanksgiving Journal to record what you are thankful for today.

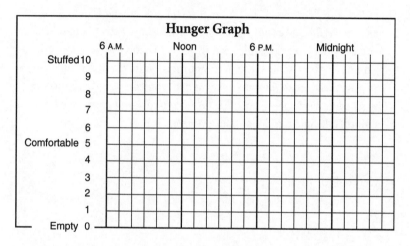

Hunger Graph

Thin Within **Food Log**

Hunger # before Eating	Time	Items/Amount	Hunger # after Eating

Thin Within Observations and Corrections Chart—Day 27

Observations	Day 27
1. I ate when my body was hungry.	
2. I ate in a calm environment by reducing distractions.	
3. I ate when I was sitting.	
4. I ate when my body and mind were relaxed.	
5. I ate and drank the things my body enjoyed.	
6. I paid attention to my food while eating.	
7. I ate slowly, savoring each bite.	
8. I stopped before my body was full.	

Gratitude List

_____

_____

_____

Thin Within Wisdom

Invite the Lord into your weariness and He will give you rest and peace.

NOTE
1. Our thanks to Bev Bradley for giving a devotional on this subject in Sacramento, California. Much of what she shared in a thirty minute talk we have adapted for Days Twenty-Seven and Twenty-Eight.

꧁

Complete In His Tenderness: Part 2

This is what the LORD says:
"Stand at the crossroads and look;
ask for the ancient paths, ask where the good way is,
and walk in it, and you will find rest for your souls.
But you said, 'We will not walk in it.'"
—Jeremiah 6:16

So many hills and valleys have been crossed during your journey. Your faithfulness to the Lord over these past four weeks has been a tribute to the grace of God at work in Your heart. The godly choices you make will infuse your life with greater joy and peace.

Long after this Thin Within adventure is over, we hope that you will continue to walk on the path of God's provision, which leads to holiness and wholeness in Christ. Your experiences over the past twenty-seven days and your life in Him affirm His faithfulness. Today we will continue to focus your attention on the "rest" that Christ promises us when we come to Him.

Come to me, all you who are weary and burdened, and I will give you rest.
Take my yoke upon you and learn from me, for I am gentle and humble in
heart, and you will find rest for your souls. For my yoke is easy and my burden
is light (Matthew 11:28–30).

How can we experience the rest Christ promises in the midst of our busy and bustling lives? The above passage speaks to that question.

1. By coming to Him when He calls. In the quietness of prayer, in obedient choices, in the weeping of repentant tears.

2. By admitting that we are weary and burdened. Christ knows our condition and He has the answer. We confess our plight through prayer and we confirm our confession when we stop striving in our own strength.

3. By bowing our heads and willingly placing them in His yoke. It is up to us to surrender our rights, our choices, our schedules, our willful spirits, our need to please others, our need to perform; to see all and be all.

4. By learning from Him.

Consider the image that Christ has painted with His words.

Take my yoke upon you and learn from me (Matthew 11:29a).

What is a yoke? According to *Harper's Bible Dictionary*, it is "a wooden or iron frame for joining two oxen or other draft animals so they can pull a plow, cart, or other heavy load. A yoke generally consisted of a single crossbar with leather or rope nooses or wooden rods that were fastened around the animals' necks. The crossbar was attached to a shaft that pulled the load."[1]

A yoke was used figuratively as a symbol of hardship, submission, or servitude. Jeremiah wore a yoke to symbolize his message that Judah should submit to Babylon (Jeremiah 27–28). When the people of Israel considered whether or not they would accept Rehoboam as king, they asked him to lighten the heavy yoke, i.e., the hard service, that his father, Solomon, imposed on them (1 Kings 12:1–11). A yoke may refer to other burdens or responsibilities, such as sin (Lamentations 1:14), service to God (Lamentations 3:27; Jeremiah 2:20; 5:5), slavery (Exodus 6:6), or obedience to Torah (Acts 15:10) or Christ (Matthew 11:29–30).

To submit willingly to a yoke is to submit to the authority of the one to whom we are bound. As Beth Moore, author and Bible teacher, states, "There is no such thing as yoke-free living."[2] We will bow to someone or something. Jesus is requesting that we offer ourselves in surrender to Him and His call. Thankfully, unlike the yokes of slavery, the law, or hard service, Jesus promised that His yoke would be easy and that His burden would be light. In fact, He promised to be our yoke-fellow, the one who would pull alongside us and bear much of the burden.

When He talks about His yoke, He reinforces the principle that to submit to Him brings peace. Submitting to authority is never easy in our fleshly state. However, the Lord, as we have seen, is just, good, gracious, kind, faithful, loving, unchanging, compassionate, powerful, and so much more. He has only our sincere needs and interests at heart, and His authority is one to which we can gladly bow. It is in submitting to one so good and powerful and loving that we find peace and rest.

Yesterday we spoke of three reasons that we may become weary.

1. We invest ourselves in things not part of God's plan.
2. We invest ourselves in godly activities beyond God's plan.
3. We invest in our own strength rather than His in doing what God calls us to do.

Today we would like to introduce one more reason for weariness:

We procrastinate doing that which God does call us to do.

The Greek word *anapausis*, translated "rest" in the passage from Matthew 11, means "rest, inward tranquility while one performs necessary labor."[3]

Cassandra has a disordered home that is a constant reminder to her that she needs to organize and clean. She is having trouble getting started and feels the burden and stress of having a huge project hanging over her head, knowing that her disordered environment affects her ability to function. She doesn't even have a suitable place to eat, which contributes to chaotic eating. Each time she walks through the door, the mess greets her and shouts an accusation, "You are a lazy bum!"

Cassandra's club of condemnation is beating her into the ground. She doesn't know how she can find the time to do all that she has to do, yet she spends untold time and energy worrying and fretting about it. Meanwhile she retreats into evening television shows to anesthetize the anxiety she has about this area of her life.

Does this sound like a life of peace and joy? Absolutely not. Cassandra prayerfully evaluated her daily activities and removed everything from her schedule that God hadn't called her to do. She found that there most certainly was some available time. Also, by eating 0 to 5, Cassandra easily freed up an extra twenty to sixty minutes a day since she is spending less time preparing or eating as much food as previously. Cassandra can now invest those minutes toward her decluttering project. Let's consider what she can accomplish.

Sunday, Cassandra, begrudgingly perhaps, spends twenty minutes in the living room. In that short amount of time, she picks up and sorts or throws away all of the magazines and newspapers that have accumulated in the living room.

Monday, feeling more optimistic, she spends twenty minutes on the entryway. Coats are hung up in the hall closet and shoes put back in bedroom closets, providing a dramatic change in this part of her house. Things don't look nearly so bad. Cassandra thinks she just might be able to have company over again sometime.

Tuesday, Cassandra is filled with energy and excitement about how much can be accomplished in so little time, she attacks the kitchen, reclaiming more "land" for the Lord and for her own sanity. In short order, she tosses the accumulated junk mail into the trash and discovers that there really is a counter underneath it all. She puts away appliances that are rarely used.

And in the last five minutes, she rejoices at the shine in her kitchen as she wipes down the counters. *Maybe I can host a Bible study later this year,* she thinks.

Wednesday she faces the family room,

Thursday, she attacks the dining room, and then continues through every room in the house until it has been transformed.

In just twenty minutes a day, Cassandra stopped stewing, and actually found herself energized by doing that to which she was called. Since that first week's activity, by investing just a few minutes each day, Cassandra can keep the bathrooms clean, the laundry done, and control the accumulation of clutter. This gives her an attitude of rest, peace, satisfaction and joy, that "feeling of inner tranquility while doing the necessary labor," as she submits to the yoke of Jesus.

Could this sort of transformation happen for you?

Take Action

Fill in the following list. Ask the Lord to join you in this activity. He might nudge you to consider things that you would otherwise overlook.

Things about Which I Procrastinate:

1. _____

2. _____

3. _____

4. _____

5. _____

6. _____

7. _____

8. _____

9. _____

10. _____

Ask God to show you which of the things you have listed is in His plan for you.

✦ Put a mark next to those things that you know God wants you to do.
A choice is before you in this very moment. If you are unsure, ask.
*Ask where the good way is, and walk in it, and you will find rest for your
souls. But you said, "We will not walk in it"* (Jeremiah 6:16b).

Unlike the people in Jeremiah's day, we hope that you will bow your head
and submit to the yoke of Christ. His yoke is easy and His burden is light.
In fact, if you are weary, it may very well be because the Spirit of God is letting you know about something that has been left undone. When we are not
in accord with our Maker, we will find ourselves weary, worn down, anxious, depressed, or stressed. But when we cooperate with Him and His plan
for us, we are energized. There is nothing more blessed than to walk in the
good works, which God prepared in advance for us to do (Ephesians 2:10).

Look at the second schedule that you set yesterday and see where you can
insert each of the marked items from today's list. As you contemplate adding
these things to your schedule, you might want to consider Cassandra's experience. She didn't try to declutter her house in a single effort, but accomplished it in twenty-minute blocks as part of her daily routine.

All that remains on the second schedule from yesterday are items that
you know God has called you to do. Anything else is off your schedule. Your
calendar now reflects, hour by hour, a life that has been willingly submitted
to the yoke of Christ.

If you have a diary or a Day-Timer for keeping track of your activities,
please update it with your new, God-given schedule. If you don't, consider
getting one for recording the schedule you have just completed. Even before
you get out of bed, it is an opportune time to start your day with prayer:
*"Lord, Let each moment of this day be lived for You and Your glory and by Your
strength only. Guide and direct my steps. Amen."*

Chuck Swindoll thinks of putting on the yoke of Christ this way:

> When I put my clothes on I want to think of it as putting a yoke on
> that belongs to you and is going to link us together.
>
> I deliberately release the cares of my day to you. I know there are
> going to be pressures, demands, stresses but they are not mine, they
> are yours. You are the stronger of these two oxen. I want to walk in
> your strength, I want to give the pressure to you, to relax and to retreat
> to your power and care and I want to abide in Christ deliberately.[4]

Is it necessary to have every minute of your schedule blocked off?

We hope you haven't done that. You will need time to smell the roses and love your neighbors. You see, rest involves just that . . . rest. Not only will we experience our hearts being at rest when our schedules are filtered through God's loving hands, but there will also be time to break free of the constraints of a rigid schedule.

✦ Look over your schedule again to be certain that you have allowed time for rest. Make the necessary adjustments.

✦ Consider this:

Then, because so many people were coming and going that they did not even have a chance to eat, he said to them, "Come with me by yourselves to a quiet place and get some rest." So they went away by themselves in a boat to a solitary place (Mark 6:31–32).

Why the need for a solitary place? *"Because so many people were coming and going . . ."* And *"they did not even have a chance to eat."* These guys were busy. The disciples lived life on the go for three years. They traveled around constantly, healing, casting out demons, teaching, being taught, ministering, managing. It was a life of busy-ness, but their schedules reflected God's plan. They undoubtedly experienced the peace and joy of living surrendered lives. Even so, Jesus advised them to break away for quiet, for rest, for time alone.

God's will is for you to rest, to have a chance to "re-create." As Beth Moore states in her Breaking Free series, there is a place for quiet where our goal is nothing but being refreshed and re-created in Him. In that place we don't need to pray for the cares of the world, which will be there when we return. We don't need to study our Bible, the truth of which will endure forever. In that place, we are to *Be still, and know that I am God* (Psalm 46:10a).

We are to have fun, laugh, enjoy and to do so blessedly knowing that He has called us to it. And we are to do it free from guilt. Remember that on the seventh day following six days of intense creativity and work, even God rested—not because He was tired, but to contemplate and enjoy the magnificence of His creation. We, who have been created in His image, need to do the same. It is ordained by God, and He blesses the weary one who rests in Him.

List below what you might enjoy doing during those moments when Jesus calls you away to a solitary place. It may be something like sitting on a quiet beach, walking through a park, skydiving, or visiting art galleries. Ask the Lord to show you. It can be something fun. Something inspiring. Something that infuses your life with joy.

What Are Some Things I Could Do to Relax?

1. _____

2. _____

3. _____

4. _____

Ask the Lord if there is a time in the upcoming week when you could enjoy one or more of these activities. As He directs you, place it on your updated schedule.

Jesus still speaks to us:

I will give you rest.

I am gentle.

I am humble.

You will find rest.

My yoke is easy.

And My burden is light.

When we are yoked with Christ, we are on the blessed path of God's provision that leads to the holy life. It is a life made whole by the gracious hand of our Savior. As this process is unfolding, we are enabled, again by God's grace, to love others and to love God as He so desires. We are living in that authentic place where we experience His rest, abundance, and provision. Our lives yield fruit when our hearts overflow with bounty that is clearly not from ourselves, but ever and always from Him, because of Him, and unto Him.

Your Success Story

Any new insights while you were reading today?

_____

_____

_____

Verses to Ponder

He gives strength to the weary and increases the power of the weak (Isaiah 40:29).

I will refresh the weary and satisfy the faint (Jeremiah 31:25).

We continually remember before our God and Father your work produced by faith, your labor prompted by love, and your endurance inspired by hope in our Lord Jesus Christ (1 Thessalonians 1:3).

For we are God's workmanship, created in Christ Jesus to do good works, which God prepared in advance for us to do (Ephesians 2:10).

Prayer

Lord, please let my schedule reflect only things that You have called me to do. I pray that I will submit to Your yoke as You lead me in the way I should go. Help me to surrender to You and allow You to have your way with my time and with everything I do. In Christ's name, Amen.

Medical Moment

Chronic sustained stress, anxiety, and tension are almost the by-words of our present life and probably cause or contribute to most of the physical and psychological ills of modern people. Sadly many of these burdens are self-imposed, resulting from the way we view ourselves and our relationship to the world around us. I once heard a story about a man who sought out the Lord. He complained that his cross was too heavy to bear. The Lord took the man's cross and directed him to a nearby room where he would be able to choose a more suitable cross. On entering the room the man was amazed to find thousands and thousands of crosses—all sizes and shapes. He searched and searched, carefully avoiding the large heavy crosses, until he found the smallest of all in a far corner of the room. Pleased that he found one so light, he returned with it to the Lord, who said to him, "The cross you chose is identical to the one you first brought to Me."

It is important that we not overburden ourselves with concerns and frustrations that we could share with the Lord.

The focus of Days Twenty-Seven and Twenty-Eight has been to point out the importance of rest. It is only with the Lord's strength and the guidance of the Holy Spirit that our yoke can be lightened, making us more faithful and healthier servants for His purposes.

—Arthur Halliday, M.D.

Success Tools

- ✦ Fill in the Hunger Graph.
- ✦ Fill in the Thin Within Food Log.
- ✦ Mark the Thin Within Observations and Corrections Chart for today.
- ✦ Use the Thin Within Keys to Conscious Eating.
- ✦ Use the Gratitude List or your Thanksgiving Journal to record what you are thankful for today.

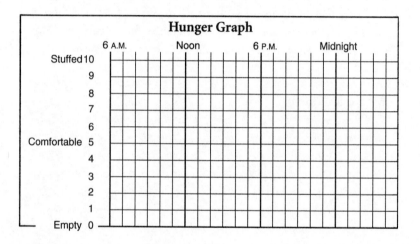

Thin Within Food Log

Hunger # before Eating	Time	Items/Amount	Hunger # after Eating

Thin Within Observations and Corrections Chart—Day 28

Observations	Day 28
1. I ate when my body was hungry.	
2. I ate in a calm environment by reducing distractions.	
3. I ate when I was sitting.	
4. I ate when my body and mind were relaxed.	
5. I ate and drank the things my body enjoyed.	
6. I paid attention to my food while eating.	
7. I ate slowly, savoring each bite.	
8. I stopped before my body was full.	

Gratitude List

_____

_____

_____

Thin Within Wisdom

To get back on the path of God's provision, ask Him for wisdom. His way will give you peace and rest. It is that easy!

NOTES
1. *Harper's Bible Dictionary*, s.v. "yoke" (New York, New York: Harper and Row, 1985), 1153.
2. Beth Moore, *Breaking Free Video Series*, video session 7, 60 minutes, Lifeway, 1999.
3. ibid. Used by permission.
4. From "Resting in Christ" (tape number MGS-4A), by Charles R. Swindoll, copyright 1999. Published by Insight for Living, Plano, TX 75026. All rights reserved. Used by permission.

Remaining Steadfast in His Embrace

*Let us not give up meeting together, as some are in the habit of doing,
but let us encourage one another—and all the more
as you see the Day approaching.*
—Hebrews 10:25

After journeying together for nearly a month, we are able to review the results of our efforts. The walls providing boundary lines for our temple have been completed. In the clear light of day the temple stands restored, bearing witness to hours spent in prayer and study, to hard work and obedience.

Every good and perfect gift is from above, coming down from the Father of the heavenly lights, who does not change like shifting shadows (James 1:17).

No one but God could have worked such change in your heart. And now that you have been restored, we rest in the knowledge that each of us really is a temple for His glory. Our bodies, our schedules, our affections, our very lives are not our own. We have been bought at a price. We affirm again that we gladly submit to the yoke of Christ, because we've learned that to do so gives us peace, rest, and abundant joy.

After Nehemiah and the faithful Israelites had completed the restoring and rebuilding of the walls around Jerusalem (Nehemiah 1–7), life didn't continue just as before. You see, the work wasn't complete merely because the physical walls were in place. Lives had to be rebuilt as well, so Nehemiah turned his attention to his people.

The strategy he used began with instruction in God's Word through Ezra, the priest. Let's see what happened during their first "Bible study."

Ezra opened the book. All the people could see him because he was standing above them; and as he opened it, the people all stood up. Ezra praised the LORD, *the great God; and all the people lifted their hands and responded, "Amen! Amen!" Then they bowed down and worshiped the* LORD *with their faces to the ground. The Levites . . . instructed the people in the Law while the people were standing there. They read from the Book of the Law of God, mak-*

ing it clear and giving the meaning so that the people could understand what was being read (Nehemiah 8:5–8).

This passage explains how God's people turned to Him after the completion of their building project. The first important observation is as follows.

1. People were in community.

You have come a long way in participating in the rebuilding process. We commend you for your diligence and perseverance. If you are not connected with a Thin Within support group, you probably have done the major reconstruction work on your own in the presence of the Lord. However, we were created in the image of God who exists as three persons in one, the most intimate relationship ever, and we were designed for relationships, for community.

Where are you in terms of your involvement regarding community? Where do you get together with others to share support?

_____

_____

_____

_____

+ Do these community opportunities include support for you specifically in your efforts with Thin Within? Yes ___ No___
+ Could you find or create an opportunity for community with regard to Thin Within? Thin Within is a *lifestyle* that continues after you close this book. How can you offer or receive support in this lifestyle?

_____

_____

_____

_____

For we are the temple of the living God (2 Corinthians 6:16).

Consequently, you are no longer foreigners and aliens, but fellow citizens with God's people and members of God's household, built on the foundation of the apostles and prophets, with Christ Jesus himself as the chief cornerstone. In him the whole building is joined together and rises to become a holy temple in the Lord. And in him you too are being built together to become a dwelling in which God lives by his Spirit (Ephesians 2:19–22).

We have learned that each of us is a temple of the Holy Spirit. But Paul expands that concept in this passage from Ephesians. He explains that believers together comprise His temple. That is another reason it is important for you to be involved in a Christian community of other people who love and support you, as well as offer accountability and prayer.

There is a second observation we can glean from the Nehemiah 8:5–8 passage.

2. People prayed.

Throughout our journey we have encouraged you to talk to God. On Day Fifteen we highlighted the value of conversing with God throughout the day. Prayer is talking honestly to God and listening to Him as well. As your Savior and Lord, He isn't silent. He longs to hear your heart and to minister to your soul.

3. People worshiped.

"A world can be set on fire by a heart set free."[1] It is our prayer that you have been set free during the past twenty-eight days to live the surrendered abundant life. When a person is set free, the only authentic response is to fall down in worship. The Israelites who stood within the secured walls of God's city had known exile and now they knew freedom. They knew hard work and they wanted to acknowledge God's inspiration and provision. Their response was eager, heart-felt worship. What are the differences between everyday worship and the worship of those who find themselves set free? The following points on authentic worship are adapted from a message given by Pastor Greg Krieger at Bayside Church:

1. Authentic worshipers discover the true God.

If a person experiences the pardon, provision, presence, and power of God in their lives, they have seen the true God. They acknowledge Him as the Creator who cannot be understood fully by the created. He is *God.*

2. Authentic worshipers see themselves clearly.

When we capture a proper vision of perfection, we realize instantly that we are far from perfect. Consider Nehemiah 8:9:

For all the people had been weeping as they listened to the words of the Law.

As the people heard the law (or Torah) being read they began to weep. They were aware of their own imperfection. Before holy God, authentic worshipers see their unholiness and recognize their need of a God of grace.

3. Authentic worshipers experience absolute healing.

As deep as runs our confusion, so much deeper runs His peace.

As deep as runs our pain, so much deeper runs His love.

As deep as runs our sin, so much deeper runs His forgiveness.

As deep as runs our brokenness, so much deeper runs His healing.

As you worship God in response to His grace, we hope your healing has been genuine and deep, and that it continues. Consider Nehemiah 8:12:

Then all the people went away to eat and drink, to send portions of food and to celebrate with great joy, because they now understood the words that had been made known to them.

4. *Authentic worshipers become agents of change in God's spiritual revolution.*

Pastor Greg Krieger stated in his message on authentic worship that once God's grace happens *to* you, it can't help but to happen *through* you. And this takes us back to community. You won't want to be in isolation for long if you have experienced the transforming power of the grace of God. It must be freely shared.[2]

No one lights a lamp and hides it in a jar or puts it under a bed. Instead, he puts it on a stand, so that those who come in can see the light (Luke 8:16).

There is simply no way that we can hide this light in a jar. Let it shine. Give glory to your Lord and Maker.

Take Action

Let's see how far you have come since the beginning of your journey together. Below you will find the questionnaire that you first completed in the "Before You Begin" section of the book. We encourage you to answer the questions again even though some of your answers may be the same. Once you are finished, compare your answers with those on the first survey.

Where I've Come From

On the following questions, circle the number that best applies: (We are starting at question number six because 1–5 are not comparative questions.)

6. How much of the time are you on a diet or sacrificing certain types of foods?

1	2	3	4	5	6	7	8	9	10
Always									Never

7. How frequently do you eat foods you really enjoy?

1	2	3	4	5	6	7	8	9	10
Always									Never

8. How often do you think of yourself as a thin person?

1	2	3	4	5	6	7	8	9	10
Always									Never

9. Can you visualize or imagine yourself at your natural size—the size God designed you to be?

1	2	3	4	5	6	7	8	9	10
Always									Never

10. Do you think you are aware of your body's hunger and fullness signals?

1	2	3	4	5	6	7	8	9	10
Always									Never

Imagine that you had a fuel gauge for your stomach, much like that on a car, which registered how empty or full you were:

11. At what point on the gauge do you usually start eating?

0	1	2	3	4	5	6	7	8	9	10
Empty					Comfy					Stuffed

12. At what point on the gauge do you usually stop eating?

0	1	2	3	4	5	6	7	8	9	10
Empty					Comfy					Stuffed

What are your current concerns? Rate each item listed below.

13. Spending too much time worrying about my weight or eating behavior

0	1	2	3	4	5	6	7	8	9	10
Serious Problem									No Problem

14. Weighing frequently

0	1	2	3	4	5	6	7	8	9	10
Serious Problem									No Problem

15. Anorexia Nervosa

0	1	2	3	4	5	6	7	8	9	10
Serious Problem									No Problem

16. Bulimia

0	1	2	3	4	5	6	7	8	9	10
Serious Problem									No Problem

17. Disliking my body

0	1	2	3	4	5	6	7	8	9	10
Serious Problem									No Problem

18. Thinking too much about food

| 0 | 1 | 2 | 3 | 4 | 5 | 6 | 7 | 8 | 9 | 10 |
Serious Problem   No Problem

19. Snacking (between meals or at night)

0 1 2 3 4 5 6 7 8 9 10
Serious Problem   No Problem

20. Alcoholic beverages

0 1 2 3 4 5 6 7 8 9 10
Serious Problem   No Problem

21. Cigarettes

0 1 2 3 4 5 6 7 8 9 10
Serious Problem   No Problem

22. Feeling guilty about what I eat

0 1 2 3 4 5 6 7 8 9 10
Serious Problem   No Problem

23. Not caring at all about what I eat

0 1 2 3 4 5 6 7 8 9 10
Serious Problem   No Problem

24. Eating out of stress or boredom

0 1 2 3 4 5 6 7 8 9 10
Serious Problem   No Problem

25. Social eating (parties, restaurants)

0 1 2 3 4 5 6 7 8 9 10
Serious Problem   No Problem

In general, how do you rate your life in the following areas?

26. Health

1 2 3 4 5 6 7 8 9 10
Poor   Excellent

27. Energy level

0 1 2 3 4 5 6 7 8 9 10
Low   High

28. Physical activity

0 1 2 3 4 5 6 7 8 9 10
Sedentary   Extremely Active

29. Productivity

0	1	2	3	4	5	6	7	8	9	10
Low										High

30. Job satisfaction (consider student or housewife as a job)

0	1	2	3	4	5	6	7	8	9	10
Unsatisfying									Very Satisfying	

31. Close relationships (friends)

0	1	2	3	4	5	6	7	8	9	10
Unsatisfying									Very Satisfying	

32. Family relationships

0	1	2	3	4	5	6	7	8	9	10
Unsatisfying									Very Satisfying	

33. Sex life

0	1	2	3	4	5	6	7	8	9	10
Unsatisfying									Very Satisfying	

34. Ability to speak up for what I want

0	1	2	3	4	5	6	7	8	9	10
Difficult										Easy

35. Level of self-esteem

0	1	2	3	4	5	6	7	8	9	10
Low										High

✦ Now compare today's answers with those on your first questionnaire which will be found in the section called "Before You Begin." When you are finished, record your thoughts regarding the differences and similarities that you observe. Ask God to give you insight to see where healing and wholeness have taken place and where there is room for improvement. Is yours a heart and a body that has been set free?

_____

_____

_____

✦ You have worked long and hard. You have steadfastly persevered through trials, challenges, upheavals, joys, successes, and victories. Take a moment to praise the Lord as the Israelites did for the way in which He has worked. Write out your praise to Him here.

_____

_____

_____

✦ What verse has encouraged or inspired you the most during these twenty-nine days? Write it here.

_____

_____

_____

Following the rebuilding of the walls around God's holy city, more revival came to the hearts of the people. A deliberate purging of sin from their lives followed the reading of the Word. God's people chose to walk in obedience. On Day Twenty-Six, if you wrote a "good-bye letter," you did that very thing. You also obeyed God's voice on Days Twenty-Seven and Twenty-Eight if you adjusted your schedule. In so many ways you are like those builders of old during Nehemiah's leadership. You, like them, have made a binding agreement with God.

"In view of all this, we are making a binding agreement, putting it in writing, and our leaders, our Levites and our priests are affixing their seals to it" (Nehemiah 9:38).

One of the primary components to this covenant, or binding agreement, said,

"We will not neglect the house of our God" (Nehemiah 10:39b).

Praise God for your dedication and your perseverance. You have surrendered yourself to the Lord God. You have not neglected your body and spirit, the "house" or temple of God. You are His, bought with a price. The glory of the Lord shines forth from you. The life you live is lived in the presence of Jesus.

Your Success Story

Did you have any new insights while you were reading today? Please record them below.

_____

_____

_____

Verses to Ponder

"Stand up and praise the LORD your God, who is from everlasting to ever-
lasting. Blessed be your glorious name, and may it be exalted above all blessing
and praise. You alone are the LORD. You made the heavens, even the highest
heavens, and all their starry host, the earth and all that is on it, the seas and
all that is in them. You give life to everything, and the multitudes of heaven
worship you" (Nehemiah 9:5b, 6).

Ascribe to the LORD, O mighty ones, ascribe to the LORD glory and strength.
Ascribe to the LORD the glory due his name; worship the LORD in the splendor
of his holiness (Psalm 29:1–2).

A time is coming and has now come when the true worshipers will worship
the Father in spirit and truth, for they are the kind of worshipers the Father
seeks. God is spirit, and his worshipers must worship in spirit and in truth
(John 4:23–24).

Prayer

O, Lord, I pray that I will become a part of a community of people who
support each other and reflect Your glory. Help me experience and under-
stand more fully the truth and wisdom of Your Word. I have received so
much healing over these twenty-nine days, and I give You all the praise.
Please equip me to share Your Word and my love with others as I worship
You in Spirit and in truth, Lord. In Jesus' name, Amen.

Medical Moment

After man had been created, God said, "It is not good for man to be alone. I will make a helper suitable for him, and the Lord God made woman." There is overwhelming scientific and anecdotal evidence that we are designed for relationships, from birth to death. Babies deprived of proper mothering suffer both physically and emotionally. Maturation during the adolescent years can be profoundly affected by success, or lack of success, in relationships. Our productive years obviously depend on how we will relate to our family and to society. And we are particularly vulnerable to isolation in our final years. During the years I worked in a San Francisco AIDS clinic, I frequently was told, "I'm not afraid to die, but I'm afraid to die alone." We're not all destined to be married, but we are all meant to fulfill God's plan in our lives, and that involves others. The Great Commission (Matthew 28:18–20) proclaims that we are to "go and make disciples of all nations." This begins by each of us loving one another as He first loved us.

—ARTHUR HALLIDAY, M.D.

Success Tools

+ Fill in the Hunger Graph.
+ Fill in the Thin Within Food Log.
+ Use the Thin Within Observations and Corrections Chart for today.
+ Use the Thin Within Keys to Conscious Eating.
+ Use the Gratitude List or your Thanksgiving Journal to record what you are thankful for today.

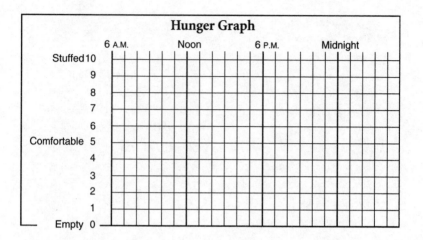

Thin Within Food Log

Hunger # before Eating	Time	Items/Amount	Hunger # after Eating

Thin Within Observations and Corrections Chart—Day 29

Observations	Day 29
1. I ate when my body was hungry.	
2. I ate in a calm environment by reducing distractions.	
3. I ate when I was sitting.	
4. I ate when my body and mind were relaxed.	
5. I ate and drank the things my body enjoyed.	
6. I paid attention to my food while eating.	
7. I ate slowly, savoring each bite.	
8. I stopped before my body was full.	

Gratitude List

_____

_____

_____

Thin Within Wisdom

Life is a wonderful journey. We continue to travel with the Lord as we hold on to His hand and He leads the way.

NOTES
1. Information and ideas on worship were inspired by a sermon message given by Pastor Greg Krieger in September, 2001, at Bayside Covenant Church in Granite Bay, California.
2. ibid.

Celebration!

Sing to the LORD a new song; sing to the LORD, all the earth.
Sing to the LORD, praise his name; proclaim his salvation day after day.
Declare his glory among the nations, his marvelous deeds among all peoples.
For great is the LORD and most worthy of praise; . . .
Splendor and majesty are before him;
strength and glory are in his sanctuary.
—Psalm 96:1–4a, 6

The sanctuary of our God now rises, splendid and majestic before His eyes. With love He looks upon you, not because of what you have done during our building process, but because He has determined, by His grace, that it is to be so. His strength and glory emanate from you, His sanctuary, His dwelling place on earth.

From a vantage point high atop the hill on which we have built, let us take a look back over the path we have traveled. The road that stretched before you on Day One as an endless trek marked by twisting turns and daunting obstacles, now lays as vanquished ground. With God's help you have conquered the land. The giants that resided there proved no match for your great God and Regal Warrior!

Today your temple is built and firmly established, secure within the restored and reinforced walls. Each reading of God's Word acts as a watchman on those walls, as a sentry guarding and preserving your newfound freedom. Your every prayer touches eternity, bridging the gap between heaven and earth, touching the heart of God.

Today we celebrate together all that God has done in you and for you. His grace continues to cascade over you, and His presence and power are guaranteed for the days ahead.

You will soon turn the last page of this book. We hope you will *not* consider this the end but a new beginning. By God's grace you are now prepared in all seasons to give a reason for the hope that lies within you (1 Peter 3:15). In fact we pray that hope is revealed in your countenance and that your face glows with the joy of new found freedom in the Lord.

Now the Lord is the Spirit, and where the Spirit of the Lord is, there is free-dom. And we, who with unveiled faces all reflect the Lord's glory, are being transformed into his likeness with ever-increasing glory, which comes from the Lord, who is the Spirit (2 Corinthians 3:17–18).

Much of our journey together has been spent getting better acquainted with the one with whom we travel. We have savored God's word and have spent time conversing with Him in prayer. We hope that throughout this restoration process you have become more intimate with the Lover of your soul.

Take Action

To see just how far you have come, we encourage you to once again com-plete the "My Relationship with God and My Relationship with Myself" Questionnaire. You first answered these questions on Day Two. It is our prayer that the miles you have logged and the progress you have made on our journey will be reflected in your new responses. (Please wait to compare your two questionnaires until you have finished the second one.)

My Relationship with God and My Relationship with Myself

After the following questions, circle the number that best applies.

1. I am comfortable with myself and my personality.

1	2	3	4	5	6	7	8	9	10
Never									Always

2. I am optimistic that I can change.

1	2	3	4	5	6	7	8	9	10
Never									Always

3. I have a tendency to put myself down or to call myself names.

1	2	3	4	5	6	7	8	9	10
Never									Always

4. I try to make others happy and to meet their expectations of me.

1	2	3	4	5	6	7	8	9	10
Never									Always

5. I derail my own goals.

1	2	3	4	5	6	7	8	9	10
Never									Always

6. I am self-conscious.

1   2   3   4   5   6   7   8   9   10
Never   Always

7. I feel I deserve to be put down by others.

1   2   3   4   5   6   7   8   9   10
Never   Always

8. My heart feels empty.

1   2   3   4   5   6   7   8   9   10
Never   Always

9. God is pleased with me.

1   2   3   4   5   6   7   8   9   10
Never   Always

10. I am angry at God.

1   2   3   4   5   6   7   8   9   10
Never   Always

11. I feel that God is angry with me.

1   2   3   4   5   6   7   8   9   10
Never   Always

12. God cares about how I feel.

1   2   3   4   5   6   7   8   9   10
Never   Always

13. I feel that God is reliable and trustworthy in my life.

1   2   3   4   5   6   7   8   9   10
Never   Always

14. I fear releasing my life completely to God.

1   2   3   4   5   6   7   8   9   10
Never   Always

15. God seems so distant.

1   2   3   4   5   6   7   8   9   10
Never   Always

16. I think God cares about my body and food issues.

1   2   3   4   5   6   7   8   9   10
Never   Always

17. I know God is there when I pray.

1	2	3	4	5	6	7	8	9	10
Never									Always

18. I think God forgives me.

1	2	3	4	5	6	7	8	9	10
Never									Always

19. I feel that I can confide in God.

1	2	3	4	5	6	7	8	9	10
Never									Always

20. I am aware of how God sees me, and I live my life accordingly.

1	2	3	4	5	6	7	8	9	10
Never									Always

21. I feel accepted and loved unconditionally by God.

1	2	3	4	5	6	7	8	9	10
Never									Always

22. I enjoy experiencing God's presence when I pray.

1	2	3	4	5	6	7	8	9	10
Never									Always

Now comes the best part. Compare this survey with the one that you took on Day Two. Note the similarities and differences.

♦ How has your view of yourself changed since you began this journey?

_____

_____

_____

♦ How has your view of God changed since you began this journey?

_____

_____

_____

♦ List below anything that you have learned or ways in which you have grown in the past thirty days, i.e., anything that you have not mentioned in the spaces above.

_____

_____

_____

_____

_____

In the days of King David, the Ark of the Covenant represented the presence of God. When David, this "man after God's heart," decided to bring the Ark into Jerusalem, something incredible happened.

So David went down and brought up the ark of God from the house of Obed-Edom to the City of David with rejoicing. . . . David, wearing a linen ephod, danced before the LORD with all his might, while he and the entire house of Israel brought up the ark of the LORD with shouts and the sound of trumpets (2 Samuel 6:12b, 14–15).

Now, as in Bible times, the presence of the Lord gives us good reason to celebrate. If our hearts are in tune with the heart of God, we will dance and shout, sing and praise Him. We hope that today is a time of joy for you. God has done so very much for all of us. Just His presence alone, in our midst, in our lives, is cause enough to rejoice.

As we part ways, we encourage you to cling tenaciously to the Savior who has bought you, the King that has wooed you, the Master that has freed you, and the Hero that has rescued you.

He has walked with you through these days and has helped you face some difficult things. You have come to rest in and appreciate the body He has given you as His creation, recognizing that you are fearfully and wonderfully made. You have embraced your identity in Christ. You have resisted reverting to the flesh and have held on to His grace. You have surrendered yourself to His yoke. You have purposely pursued the holy life. His promises have come to pass in your life. He has said to you:

"I have loved you with an everlasting love; I have drawn you with lovingkindness. I will build you up again and you will be rebuilt, O Virgin Israel. Again you will take up your tambourines and go out to dance with the joyful" (Jeremiah 31:3–4).

God has made a way in the wilderness for you to walk on the path of His provision, leading you into a life of holiness as you enjoy the abundant life.

Today is the day to take up your tambourine, to dance with joy, and to know that we will continue to pray for you and with you, lifting you up.

To him who is able to keep you from falling and to present you before his glorious presence without fault and with great joy—to the only God our Savior be glory, majesty, power and authority, through Jesus Christ our Lord, before all ages, now and forevermore. Amen (Jude 24–25).

A Note from the Authors

We love hearing from our readers. You can contact us at:

> Thin Within
> 101 First St. PMB 438
> Los Altos, CA 94022

Please also visit our author website at: www.hallidayministries.com

To learn about how you can participate in the Thin Within Program, refer to the following information from Bill Dembereckyj, the president of Thin Within.

> In the love of Christ,
> Judy and Arthur Halliday

A Note from the President

Congratulations on taking a step towards living an abundant life in Christ. I hope that your experience reading the new version of *Thin Within* has truly helped you. For many of you this is a beginning step toward reshaping your body and your soul into that which is honoring to God. For others, it is just one of many steps that you have taken down this road that will finally lead you to the results for which you have longed. Wherever you find yourself on this journey, please know that you are not alone. Millions of people around the world are accepting this challenge just like you.

It is for all of you that we have created the Thin Within organization. Thin Within is much more than a book. It is a global network of people in support groups who are seeking to embrace an abundant life and return to a natural size. It is an on-going program of weekly lessons and exercises created to challenge, motivate, and encourage you. It is a team of people who care about you and want to help you succeed in reaching your goals. Finally, it is a community of Christians working together to serve God and change lives all around the world.

All of it starts at www.ThinWithin.org. This site is your passport to finding support groups in your area, continuing your personal growth through your own Thin Within online program, interacting with others from around the world, sharing and reading stories of personal struggles and victories and much, much more. Get involved today! We look forward to hearing from you and welcoming you into our community. Please visit us at our website: **www.ThinWithin.org** or call us at 877-729-8932.

—Bill Dembereckyj
President